Multiple Cho Lecture Notes on Clinical Medicine

MW01227211

JOHN BRADLEY
BMedSci (Nottm.) MRCP BM BS
Registrar
Addenbrooke's Hospital
Cambridge

DAVID RUBENSTEIN
MA MD FRCP (Lond.)
Physician
Addenbrooke's Hospital
Cambridge

DAVID WAYNE
MA BM FRCP (Lond. & Edin.)
Physician
James Paget District Hospital
Gorleston, Great Yarmouth

THIRD EDITION

BLACKWELL SCIENTIFIC PUBLICATIONS

OXFORD LONDON EDINBURGH

BOSTON PALO ALTO MELBOURNE

© 1978, 1982, 1987 by
Blackwell Scientific Publications
Editorial offices:
Osney Mead, Oxford OX2 0EL
   (*Orders*: Tel. 0865 240201)
8 John Street, London WC1N 2ES
23 Ainslie Place, Edinburgh EH3 6AJ
52 Beacon Street, Boston
   Massachusetts 02108, USA
667 Lytton Avenue, Palo Alto
   California 94301, USA
107 Barry Street, Carlton
   Victoria 3053, Australia

First published 1978
Reprinted 1979, 1980
Second edition 1982
Reprinted 1985
Third edition 1987

Photoset by Enset (Photosetting),
Midsomer Norton, Bath, Avon
Printed and bound
in Great Britain

DISTRIBUTORS

USA
   Year Book Medical Publishers
   35 East Wacker Drive
   Chicago, Illinois 60601
   (*Orders*: Tel. 312-726-9733)

Canada
   The C.V. Mosby Company
   5240 Finch Avenue East
   Scarborough, Ontario
   (*Orders*: Tel. 416-298-1588)

Australia
   Blackwell Scientific Publications
   (Australia) Pty Ltd
   107 Barry Street
   Carlton, Victoria 3053
   (*Orders*: Tel. (03) 347-0300)

British Library
Cataloguing in Publication Data

Bradley, John
   Multiple choice questions on
   lecture notes on clinical medicine.
   — 3rd ed.
   1. Pathology — Problems,
   exercises, etc.
   I. Title   II. Rubenstein, David
   III. Wayne, David
   616'.0076   RB119

   ISBN 0-632-01816-X

Multiple Choice Questions on Lecture Notes on Clinical Medicine

CONTENTS

v

PREFACE

The chief use of multiple choice questions (MCQs) is in revision and discussion. They can sharpen a student's jaded mind — there can be no self-deceiving excuses for a wrong answer after it has been written down. Thus unrecognized lacunae in knowledge can be discovered and corrected. Accordingly, we recommend that the student answer these questions on his own by *writing out* the answers to a whole block of questions. This is preferable to looking up the answer to each question one by one after making a half-hearted mental commitment. This also avoids spoiling the next question by inadvertently spotting the answer to it. It is best to discuss with some of the answers, for they often concern matters of opinion and weighting rather than absolute truth. If you do not like the answers given you will feel more secure in your disagreement if a whole group of doctors agrees with you. If you do find any serious errors or feel that any answer is particularly bizarre, please let us know.

In this edition we have modified or replaced all the questions, and the answers are now given in extended form with discussion. We have also added a separate 60-question MCQ test paper which ideally should be attempted in a single uninterrupted session of 2½ hours.

Reading textbooks is generally very boring and we hope that these questions will add a hint of enjoyment to the grind of study. Good luck — we hope you get all of them right.

1987   John Bradley
                                            David Rubenstein
                                              David Wayne

PART ONE

1. **Bitemporal hemianopia can occur with**
    A   Temporal lobe astrocytoma
    B   Craniopharyngioma
    C   Pinealoma
    D   Internal carotid artery aneurysm
    E   Pituitary tumour

2. **Ptosis**
    A   May be present in lower motor neuron 7th nerve palsies
    B   Is usually partial following damage to the cervical sympathetic chain
    C   Occurs in myaesthenia gravis
    D   Occurs in dystrophia myotonica
    E   May be congenital

3. **A small pupil is seen in**
    A   Argyll Robertson pupils
    B   3rd nerve palsy
    C   Atropine
    D   Pilocarpine
    E   Neostigmine

1. BDE

Bitemporal hemianopia suggests chiasmal compression of the optic nerve. It is usually caused by a pituitary tumour or more rarely a craniopharyngioma (a benign congenital tumour which arises in the remnant of the craniopharyngeal duct), or an internal carotid artery aneurysm. The pineal gland lies between the superior colliculi, being attached by a stalk to the posterior wall of the third ventricle, and is thus not related to the optic nerve.

2. BCDE

The levator palpebrae superioris is supplied by the superior ramus of the oculomotor nerve. In addition smooth muscle fibres are innervated by sympathetic nerves. Ptosis occurs with 3rd nerve lesions (when it is usually complete), sympathetic lesions as part of a Horner's syndrome (when it is usually partial) or diseases causing primary muscle weakness. It may be congenital.

3. ADE

The pupillary muscles are supplied by constrictor para-sympathetic fibres, which travel from the Edinger–Westphal nucleus with the oculomotor nerve to the ciliary ganglion and thence through the short ciliary nerves to the constrictor pupillae muscle, and dilator sympathetic fibres which follow a complicated course from the brain stem to the long ciliary nerves (cf. below). Small pupils therefore result from lesions of the sympathetic nerves or from parasympathomimetic drugs. The site of the lesion in Argyll Robertson pupils (small irregular pupils which accommodate but do not react) is probably the ciliary ganglion.

4. **Horner's syndrome may occur in**
   A   Multiple sclerosis
   B   Compression of the spinal cord at the level of the 2nd thoracic vertebra
   C   Internal carotid artery aneurysms
   D   Cervical rib
   E   Pancoast's syndrome

5. **The following are typical of Horner's syndrome**
   A   Enophthalmos
   B   Anhydrosis
   C   Pupillary dilatation
   D   Ptosis
   E   Paralysis of outward gaze of the eye

6. **The ulnar nerve**
   A   Arises from the medial cord of the brachial plexus
   B   May be damaged by dislocation of the elbow
   C   Supplies the thenar eminence
   D   Causes wrist drop if compressed in the ulnar groove
   E   Causes sensory loss over the dorsum of the hand when compressed at the wrist

4. ACDE

5. ABD
The majority of the sympathetic nerves to the eye arise in the hypothalamus. Preganglionic fibres pass through the pons and medulla and exit with the anterior nerve roots of C_8 and T_1 to the superior cervical ganglion. Post-ganglionic fibres pass in the carotid sheath with the internal carotid through the cavernous sinus to join the ophthalmic branch of the trigeminal nerve. They supply the levator palpebrae superioris and dilator pupillae and cause vasodilatation and sweating in the face.

Paralysis of the sympathetic nerves at any site gives rise to Horner's syndrome which is characterized by meiosis, enophthalmos, anhydrosis and ptosis (everything gets smaller or contracts). It may occur due to vascular lesions, compression or demyelination. Pancoast's syndrome is an apical carcinoma of the bronchus giving rise to a T_1 lesion with Horner's syndrome.

6. AB
The ulnar nerve arises from the medial cord of the brachial plexus, usually with a contribution from the lateral cord ($C_{7.8}$, T_1). In the hand it supplies the hypothenar muscles, the interossei, the 3rd and 4th lumbricals, the adductor pollicis and part of the flexor pollicis brevis. It is usually damaged by compression in the ulnar groove at the elbow causing the characteristic claw hand (wrist drop is a feature of radial nerve palsy). The dorsal branch which supplies the skin over the dorsal aspect of the hand arises in the forearm and is spared by compression at the wrist.

4

7. Carpal tunnel syndrome
A   Is due to compression of the radial nerve at the wrist
B   Causes paraesthesia of the palmar surface of the little finger and half of the ring finger
C   Causes wasting of the thenar eminence
D   May occur in rheumatoid arthritis
E   May occur in chronic renal failure

8. The femoral nerve
A   Arises from the sacral plexus
B   Has contributions from the 2nd to 4th lumbar nerve roots
C   Lies medial to the femoral artery beneath the inguinal ligament
D   May be damaged by dislocation of the hip
E   If damaged causes loss of the knee jerk

9. In facial nerve palsy due to herpes zoster (Ramsay Hunt syndrome)
A   Movements of the forehead are usually retained
B   There may be an accompanying 6th nerve palsy
C   *Varicella zoster* virus can be identified in the geniculate ganglion
D   Hyperacusis occurs
E   There is loss of taste over the anterior two thirds of the tongue

7. CDE

Carpal tunnel syndrome is due to compression of the median nerve as it passes deep to the flexor retinaculum. It causes sensory loss on the palmar surface of the thumb and radial two and a half fingers, and thenar wasting with weakness of thumb abduction and opposition. In chronic renal failure it may result from arteriovenous fistula formation at the wrist or amyloid deposition in the flexor retinaculum.

8. BDE

The femoral nerve arises from the lumbar plexus (L_{2-4}). It enters the thigh behind the inguinal ligament where it lies lateral to the femoral artery. In the thigh it supplies quadriceps femoris, pectineus and sartorius and sensation to the front of the thigh. Damage usually occurs as a result of fractures of the femur or pelvis or dislocation of the hip and causes weakness of knee extension, wasting of quadriceps, loss of knee jerk and sensory impairment over the front of the thigh. The femoral nerve continues as the saphenous nerve to supply the skin over the medial aspect of the lower leg.

9. CDE

The anatomical relationships of the facial nerve enable lesions to be located accurately. Fibres to the upper facial muscles are represented in both sides of the cerebral cortex and thus movements of the forehead are retained in upper motor neuron lesions. 6th and 7th nerve palsies usually occur together with lesions in the pons due to the close proximity of their nuclei at this site. The Ramsay Hunt syndrome is due to herpes zoster of the geniculate ganglion in the tympanic cavity. The nerve to the stapedius muscle and the chorda tympani arise in the facial canal and are thus affected by lesions of the geniculate ganglion.

10. **Dysarthria occurs in**
    A Bell's palsy
    B Parkinson's disease
    C Infarction of the posterior inferior part of the dominant frontal lobe (Broca's area)
    D Bulbar palsy
    E Pseudobulbar palsy

11. **The following are features of hypermetropia**
    A Concave spectacle lenses
    B Short sightedness
    C Small optic discs on ophthalmoscopy
    D Temporal pallor of the disc
    E Absent ankle jerks

12. **Subacute combined degeneration of the cord is associated with**
    A Damage to the dorso-lateral columns
    B Absent knee jerks
    C Brisk ankle jerks
    D Diminished sensation to all modalities in the feet
    E Upgoing plantar reflexes

10. ABDE
Dysarthria is the inability to articulate properly due to paralysis or inco-ordination of the muscles involved in speech. Bulbar palsy describes lower motor neuron palsies of the 9th, 10th and 12th cranial nerves and pseudo-bulbar palsy upper motor neuron palsies. Lesions of Broca's area give rise to an expressive dysphasia.

11. C
In hypermetropia (longsightedness) the eyeball is too short and a positive lens (convex, magnifying) is required for correction. The optic disc appears small with ill defined margins. Absent tendon reflexes occur together with dilated sluggishly reacting pupils in the Holmes Adie syndrome.

12. ADE
Subacute combined degeneration of the (spinal) cord refers to combined demyelination of both pyramidal (lateral) and posterior (dorsal) columns. In addition there is usually degeneration of the peripheral nerves and brain. Although vibration and position sense are always diminished due to dorsal column loss, peripheral neuropathy usually causes diminished sensation to all modalities in addition to absent ankle jerks. Knee jerks are lost less frequently and are more commonly exaggerated with upgoing plantars due to pyramidal column involvement.

13. **The ankle jerk**
    A   Is mediated by a monosynaptic reflex
    B   Is mediated through the 4th and 5th lumbar segments of the spinal cord
    C   Is elicited by tapping the tendo calcaneus
    D   Is diminished by lesions of the sciatic nerve
    E   Is diminished by transection of the cord at L_1

14. **Positive Babinski reflexes (bilateral upgoing plantar reflexes) may occur**
    A   In multiple sclerosis
    B   In pernicious anaemia
    C   In infancy
    D   Following *grand mal* convulsion
    E   In diabetes mellitus

15. **Cataracts are associated with**
    A   Hyperparathyroidism
    B   Chloramphenicol
    C   Prednisolone
    D   Rubella
    E   Duchenne muscular dystrophy

13. ACD
Tendon reflexes are mediated by a reflex arc consisting of two neurons with one synapse between them. They are diminished or abolished by lesions interrupting either the afferent, central or efferent paths of the reflex arc and exaggerated through loss of higher inhibition by lesions of the corticospinal tracts. The ankle jerk is elicited by a blow on the tendo calcaneus and causes plantar flexion of the ankle. It is mediated through the 1st and 2nd sacral components of the sciatic nerve.

14. ABCD
The Babinski (plantar) reflex is a spinal segmental reflex mediated by the first sacral segment of the cord. Extensor plantar reflexes are often observed during sleep and deep coma from any cause, for a short time after epileptic convulsions and usually in the first year of life (before the corticospinal fibres are fully developed). In any other circumstances it indicates an organic lesion of the cortico-spinal tract.

15. CD
Cataracts may be a feature of hypoparathyroidism whereas hyperparathyroidism tends to cause corneal calcification. Steroids are a well recognized cause of cataract formation. The rubella syndrome due to maternal rubella in the first trimester of pregnancy is an important cause of congenital cataracts. Cataracts are common in dystrophia myotonica but not other forms of muscular dystrophy.

16. **Massive splenomegaly is commonly found in**
   A Infectious hepatitis
   B Pernicious anaemia
   C Myelofibrosis
   D Chronic myeloid leukaemia
   E Long standing cirrhosis

17. **Ascites may be present in**
   A Cardiac failure
   B Ovarian fibroma
   C Malnutrition
   D Nephrotic syndrome
   E Inferior vena caval obstruction

18. **Unconjugated hyperbilirubinaemia is characteristic of**
   A Gilbert's syndrome
   B Dubin–Johnson syndrome
   C Rotor syndrome
   D Haemolytic anaemia
   E Crigler–Najjar syndrome

16. CD
The two commonest causes of massive splenomegaly in the UK are chronic myeloid leukaemia and myelofibrosis. On a worldwide basis malaria, and kala-azar are also common causes. The many causes of moderately or slightly enlarged spleens include other reticuloendothelial disorders (Hodgkin's, chronic lymphatic leukaemia), infections (glandular fever, brucella, infectious hepatitis, subacute bacterial endocarditis), amyloid, storage diseases and cirrhosis.

17. ABCDE
Ascites may occur as a result of inflammatory or neoplastic lesions in the abdomen, diminished oncotic pressure due to hypoalbuminaemia (as in the nephrotic syndrome and malnutrition) or an elevated hydrostatic pressure in the hepatic sinusoids (as in inferior vena caval or hepatic vein obstruction and cardiac failure). The mechanism of ascites in Meigs' syndrome (ovarian tumour, usually benign, ascites and pleural effusion) is unknown.

18. ADE
Unconjugated hyperbilirubinaemia may result from excessive bilirubin production (as in haemolytic anaemias), reduced hepatic uptake of bilirubin (which may explain the unconjugated hyperbilirubinaemia found in Gilbert's syndrome) or reduced hepatic conjugation of bilirubin (as in Crigler–Najjar syndrome). In Dubin–Johnson and Rotor syndromes there is a congenital defect of excretion of conjugated bilirubin.

19. Jaundice with pale stools and dark urine is characteristic of
A   Infectious hepatitis
B   Carcinoma of the pancreas
C   Hepatoma
D   Primary biliary cirrhosis
E   Chlorpromazine-induced jaundice

20. An elevated serum alkaline phosphatase occurs in
A   Obstructive jaundice
B   Paget's disease
C   Osteomalacia
D   Adolescence
E   Pregnancy

21. Achalasia of the cardia
A   Is a neuromuscular disorder involving the entire oesophagus
B   May present with mediastinal widening on chest X-ray
C   Often presents with recurrent pneumonia
D   Often presents with weight loss
E   Rarely recurs after oesophageal dilatation

19. ABDE
Cholestatic jaundice may result from obstruction of the extrahepatic biliary system (as in carcinoma of the pancreas) or obstruction of intrahepatic interlobular bile ducts (as in primary biliary cirrhosis or sclerosing cholangitis). In addition, intrahepatic cholestasis may be due to a secretory failure at the level of the hepatocellular canaliculi without evidence of obstruction to flow in the bile ducts. This may occur in drug-induced jaundice and viral hepatitis.

20. ABCDE
Alkaline phosphatase is found in high levels in biliary canaliculi, osteoblasts, intestinal mucosa and placenta. Serum alkaline phosphatase is thus commonly elevated in liver disease, particularly with obstruction, bone disease or during bone growth in adolescence and during the last trimester of pregnancy.

21. ABC
In achalasia of the cardia there is a degeneration of Auerbach's plexus causing abnormal peristalsis throughout the oesophagus and a failure of relaxation of the cardia. The oesophagus may become enormously dilated and spill-over of food into the lungs commonly causes pneumonia. Weight loss is an uncommon presenting feature and is usually only mild when it occurs. Treatment is either by oesophageal dilatation or surgical oesophagomyotomy (Heller's operation), but even after treatment the oesophageal contractions remain abnormal and recurrent symptoms are common.

22. The incidence of carcinoma of the oesophagus is increased in
A Achalasia of the cardia
B Reflux oesophagitis
C Hiatus hernia
D Iron deficiency anaemia
E Tylosis

23. Rectal bleeding is a feature of
A Diverticular disease
B Viral gastroenteritis
C Campylobacter enteritis
D Crohn's colitis
E Sarcoidosis

24. Haemoptysis occurs characteristically in the following
A Tuberculosis
B Pulmonary sarcoidosis
C Bronchiectasis
D Pulmonary embolism
E Pulmonary oedema

22. ADE
The increased incidence of carcinoma of the oesophagus in patients with achalasia is probably due to stasis above the cardia. Although there is an increased incidence of malignancy in patients with oesophageal strictures due to corrosives or irradiation, there is no clear relationship with reflux oesophagitis or hiatus hernia. In the Plummer–Vinson (Patterson–Kelly–Brown) syndrome iron deficiency anaemia occurs in association with a post-cricoid web which is precancerous. Tylosis is an inherited skin disease characterized by hyperkeratosis of the soles and palms which is associated with carcinoma of the oesophagus.

23. ACD
The commonest cause of rectal bleeding is haemorrhoids or fissures but their presence does not exclude other causes. Colonic carcinoma or inflammatory bowel disease should always be considered and excluded with sigmoidoscopy and barium enema if the cause is not obvious. Infections (particularly campylobacter, shigella and amoeba), ischaemic colitis and diverticular disease are other common causes.

24. ACDE
No definite cause for haemoptysis will be found in about 40% of patients. The common clinical problem is to exclude bronchial carcinoma (or rarely other tumours) and tuberculosis. It is not uncommon in infection (pneumococcal, klebsiella, lung abscess) and bronchiectasis and is characteristic of pulmonary embolism with infarction. Cardiac conditions associated with haemoptysis are mitral stenosis and pulmonary oedema. Rarer conditions include pulmonary haemosiderosis and Goodpasture's syndrome. The possibility of a foreign body should always be considered.

25. Clubbing commonly occurs in

A Bronchiectasis
B Chronic bronchitis
C Asthma
D Fibrosing alveolitis
E Mesothelioma

26. Central cyanosis characteristically occurs with

A Over 3 g/100 ml reduced haemoglobin
B Bronchial carcinoma
C Status asthmaticus
D Anaemia
E Multiple pulmonary emboli

27. Methaemoglobinaemia may be caused by

A Aspirin
B Phenacetin
C Paracetamol
D Sulphonamides
E Primaquine

25. ADE

Clubbing is associated with diseases of the lungs, heart and abdomen. Pulmonary causes include—suppurative diseases, including bronchiectasis, lung abscess and empyema (but not uncomplicated chronic bronchitis), fibrosing alveolitis and asbestosis (but rarely other causes of pulmonary fibrosis), and malignancy, especially carcinoma of the bronchus but also pleural malignancy.

26. ACE

Cyanosis describes the blue discolouration which may be seen in the nail beds, lips and tongue and is almost always due to the presence of an excess of reduced haemoglobin due to arterial hypoxaemia. Over 3 g/100 ml of reduced haemoglobin is usually present before cyanosis occurs. Thus in anaemia, severe hypoxaemia may be present without cyanosis. Cyanosis may be peripheral due to poor circulation, or central.

27. BDE

Methaemoglobinaemia is characterized by increased quantities of haemoglobin in which the iron is oxidized from the ferrous to the ferric (Fe^{3+}) form. It is a rare cause of cyanosis. It may very rarely be congenital due to an abnormality of the haemoglobin but is more commonly acquired due to the oxidant action of certain drugs. The common causes include phenacetin, sulphonamides, primaquine and certain household or industrial substances such as aniline dyes or high nitrate levels in drinking water.

28. The third heart sound

A   Occurs in systole
B   Is always abnormal
C   Is best heard with the diaphragm of the stethoscope
D   May occur in constrictive pericarditis
E   May arise from the right ventricle

29. Pulsus paradoxus may occur in

A   Asthma
B   Left ventricular failure
C   Right ventricular failure
D   Lobar pneumonia
E   Pericardial effusion

30. A prominent 'a' wave may suggest

A   Atrial fibrillation
B   Tricuspid incompetence
C   Ventricular septal defect
D   Pulmonary stenosis
E   Pulmonary hypertension

28. DE
The third heart sound occurs just after the second sound and is associated with ventricular filling. It is low pitched and thus is best heard with the bell of the stethoscope. It is common in young people but should be regarded as abnormal after the age of 40. It is common in mitral regurgitation and may occur in constrictive pericarditis. In the absence of these two conditions it implies either right, or more commonly left, ventricular disease.

29. ACE
Pulsus paradoxus may occur in obstructive airways disease, pericardial constriction or right ventricular failure. It is an accentuation of the normal decrease in the amplitude of the arterial pulse during inspiration. In normal people this probably occurs because the capacity of the pulmonary vascular bed increases during inspiration, reducing the return of blood to the left ventricle. This is partly compensated for by an increased right ventricular output in inspiration. In obstructive airways disease the powerful inspiratory effort increases the capacity of the lung vessels further and in pericardial constriction or right ventricular failure the right ventricle is unable to compensate for the increased pulmonary vascular capacity by increasing its output.

30. DE
Prominent 'a' waves are caused by forceful right atrial contraction and imply increased resistance to blood flow from the right atrium to the right ventricle. The resistance may be at the level of the tricuspid valve (tricuspid stenosis or atresia) or there may be resistance to filling of a hypertrophied right ventricle as in pulmonary stenosis and pulmonary hypertension.

31. **Cannon waves occur in**
   A   Atrial flutter with variable block
   B   Ventricular tachycardia
   C   Complete heart block
   D   Tricuspid stenosis
   E   Nodal tachycardia

32. **In aortic coarctation**
   A   The lesion is proximal to the origin of the left sub-
        clavian artery in the majority of cases
   B   Bacterial infection rarely occurs
   C   The aortic valve is commonly bicuspid
   D   Presentation in adulthood is rare
   E   Hypertension is invariably reversed by surgery

33. **The following may complicate mitral stenosis**
   A   Atrial fibrillation
   B   Systemic embolization
   C   Recurrent chest infections
   D   Haemoptysis
   E   Hoarseness

31. BCE

Cannon waves are large jugular venous pulsations synchronous with the carotid pulse due to atrial contraction against a closed tricuspid valve. They occur whenever atrial and ventricular systoles coincide. This is intermittent in complete heart block and ventricular tachycardia. In junctional rhythms atrial and ventricular contractions are synchronous and cannon waves occur with every beat.

32. C

In 98% of patients with aortic coarctation the lesion is distal to the origin of the left subclavian artery. The aortic valve is commonly bicuspid and bacterial infection may arise either on the valve or at the site of the coarctation—antibiotic prophylaxis should therefore be employed as for valvular heart disease. The majority of patients are asymptomatic and may not present until after complications, often related to hypertension, develop. Although the blood pressure usually returns to normal if surgical correction is achieved, residual hypertension may persist, particularly in the older age group.

33. ABCDE

Atrial fibrillation commonly occurs in mitral stenosis. It is often associated with a deterioration in symptoms and greatly increases the risk of systemic embolization. Haemoptysis may be associated with pulmonary venous hypertension or pulmonary infarction (the low cardiac output predisposes to venous thrombosis). Recurrent chest infections are common, complicating the chronic pulmonary congestion. Hoarseness may result from compression of the laryngeal nerve by the enlarged atrium.

34. In rheumatic aortic stenosis
A There is a pansystolic apical murmur
B The aortic second sound is clicking in character
C There is a thrill at the base of the heart
D The pulse volume is reduced
E The apex beat may be displaced laterally

35. Megaloblasts
A Are normally present in the bone marrow
B Are found in the bone marrow in vitamin B_{12} deficiency
C Are found in the bone marrow in folate deficiency
D May be present in the peripheral blood in iron deficiency
E Have small nuclei

36. The following ECG changes are characteristic of hyperkalaemia
A Sinus bradycardia
B Exaggeration of the U wave
C Flattening or inversion of the T wave
D Widening of the QRS complex
E Lengthening of the QT interval

34. CDE

Rheumatic aortic stenosis gives rise to an ejection systolic murmur which is commonly associated with a thrill at the base of the heart. An aortic ejection click may occur immediately after the first sound if the valve is not heavily calcified (thought to be due to sharp arrest of the valve in the fully open position). If the valve is heavily calcified the aortic component of the second sound may be inaudible. The pulse is usually small in volume, slow rising and prolonged (anacrotic). With severe stenosis the apex may be displaced due to left ventricular hypertrophy.

35. BC

Megaloblasts are abnormal erythroblasts characterized by a large and inactive nucleus (maturation arrest) in a relatively hypermature, even haemoglobinized cytoplasm. They are found in the marrow and only rarely in the peripheral blood. They denote defective DNA synthesis and in clinical practice this is usually due to deficiency of B_{12} or folate. They are not present in the normal marrow.

36. AD

Hyperkalaemia depresses the initiation and conduction of cardiac impulses resulting in sinus bradycardia (eventually sinus arrest), widening of the QRS complex and peaking of the T waves. The characteristic T wave changes may be obscured if the patient has been digitalized. T wave flattening or inversion is characteristic of hypokalaemia and lengthening of the QT interval is a feature of hypocalcaemia or calcium antagonists.

37. Reticulocytes

A   Are usually present in the peripheral blood
B   Are smaller than mature red cells
C   May be used to monitor the response to treatment in pernicious anaemia
D   Are found in excess in the peripheral blood in haemolytic anaemia
E   Are found in excess in the peripheral blood following haemorrhage

38. Hypoprothrombinaemia due to vitamin K deficiency

A   Is common in obstructive jaundice
B   Occurs in vegetarians
C   May be caused by antibiotics
D   Is caused by phenindione
E   Characteristically causes petechial haemorrhages

37. ACDE

Reticulocytes are the earliest non nucleated red cells in which traces of nucleoprotein remain as fine strands. On staining with the usual haematological stains they give the whole cell a faint bluish colour, and on staining with special dyes (such as brilliant cresyl blue) a fine net like appearance is seen. They are larger than mature red cells and if present in excess may give rise to a macrocytosis. Normally only about 0.5% of red cells in the peripheral blood are reticulocytes. In conditions of rapid cell degeneration, such as after haemorrhage or haemolysis or in response to vitamin B_{12}, folate or occasionally iron, the proportion increases and may reach 40% or more.

38. ACD

The synthesis in the liver of prothrombin, together with factors VII, IX and X, requires the presence of vitamin K. Vitamin K is fat soluble and its absorption is consequently defective in obstructive jaundice. It is present in many foods, although the richest source is green vegetables. In addition vitamin K is synthesized by many bacteria and some requirements are met by absorption of vitamin K produced in the gut. This explains the hypoprothrombinaemia which may follow sterilization of the intestine by antibiotics. Inandiones (such as phenindione) and coumarins (such as warfarin) antagonize the action of vitamin K. Hypoprothrombinaemia commonly causes bruising and intramuscular haemorrhages and excessive bleeding after trauma. Petechial haemorrhages are characteristic of thrombocytopenia and capillary defects.

39. Prothrombin time

A Is a measure of the extrinsic system
B Is prolonged in haemophilia
C Is prolonged in thrombocytopenia
D Is normal in fibrinogen deficiency
E Is prolonged by coumarin

40. Thrombocytopenia

A Is invariably associated with a deficiency of megakaryocytes in the bone marrow
B Is associated with hypersplenism
C Is associated with pernicious anaemia
D Causes a prolonged bleeding time
E Causes a prolonged partial thromboplastin time

39. A E
The prothrombin time is a measurement of the effectiveness
of the extrinsic system. It is the time taken for the patient's
citrated plasma to clot when a tissue factor (brain extract) and
calcium are added. It measures deficiencies of fibrinogen,
prothrombin and factors V, VII and X and is thus prolonged
by vitamin K antagonists and fibrinogen deficiency. It is
normal in haemophiliacs and thrombocytopenia.

40. B C D
Thrombocytopenia may result from decreased production of
platelets (as in marrow aplasia or infiltration, leukaemia,
megaloblastic anaemias) or increased destruction of platelets
(as in hypersplenism or immune thrombocytopenias). Megakaryocytes are deficient in the bone marrow in the first group
of conditions but are plentiful in the second group. The bleeding time is prolonged in thrombocytopenia but coagulation
times are normal.

PART TWO

NEUROLOGY

1. **The following are characteristic of raised intracranial pressure**
    A   Marked loss of visual acuity
    B   3rd nerve palsy
    C   6th nerve palsy
    D   Herniation of the cerebellar tonsils through the tentorium cerebelli
    E   Bradycardia

2. **Migraine**
    A   Is commoner in females
    B   May be familial
    C   Usually begins in childhood
    D   May respond to ergotamine
    E   May cause cerebral infarction

3. **In subdural haematoma**
    A   Blood collects between the dura mater and periosteum of the skull
    B   There is always a history of trauma
    C   The haematoma is rarely bilateral
    D   Patients are usually middle aged
    E   Patients can usually be managed conservatively

29

1.   BCE
Visual failure occurs late in papilloedema associated with raised intracranial pressure unlike that due to optic neuritis. 6th nerve palsy may occur due to compression of the nerve as it crosses the petrous temporal bone giving rise to a 'false localizing sign' and the 3rd nerve may be compressed by herniation of the medial temporal lobe through the tentorium cerebelli. The cerebellar tonsils lie below the tentorium cerebelli and may herniate through the foramen magnum. Bradycardia is thought to be due to compression or ischaemia of the cardiac centre in the medulla oblongata.

2.   ABDE
Migraine is thought to be due to cerebral arterial spasm, during which there may be cerebral ischaemia or even infarction, followed by dilatation. Ergotamine may be successful in aborting attacks provided it is given early enough. It is commoner in females and usually begins at or shortly after puberty although an onset around the menopause is not uncommon. It may be familial.

3.   None
In subdural haematoma there is a collection of blood between the dura mater and arachnoid. It is commonest in the elderly, usually but not always, resulting from trauma which may be trivial. The haematoma is bilateral in up to 50% of cases. Surgical evacuation of the blood clot is the treatment of choice.

4. **The following are features of the lateral medullary syndrome**
    A Vertigo and vomiting
    B Palatal paralysis
    C Contralateral 3rd nerve palsy
    D Contralateral Horner's syndrome
    E Ipsilateral spinothalamic loss over the trunk

5. *Petit mal* **epilepsy**
    A Usually presents in adolescence
    B Often continues into adult life
    C Is associated with a typical EEG pattern of spike and wave complexes at 3/minute
    D Is usually associated with incontinence
    E May respond to treatment with sodium valproate

6. **In a patient suspected of suffering from multiple sclerosis the following cerebrospinal fluid findings would support the diagnosis**
    A Lymphocytosis
    B Raised protein content
    C Raised IgM on immunoelectrophoresis
    D Oligoclonal bands on immunoelectrophoresis
    E Positive VDRL reaction

4. AB

In the lateral medullary syndrome infarction of the lateral aspect of the medulla and inferior surface of the cerebellum results from occlusion of either the vertebral or posterior inferior cerebellar artery. Ipsilateral cerebellar signs are usually associated with vertigo and vomiting, and ipsilateral paralysis of the soft palate, pharynx and vocal cords results from involvement of the nucleus ambiguus. Involvement of the trigeminal nerve causes sensory loss on the face. There is ipsilateral Horner's syndrome and contralateral spino-thalamic loss on the trunk.

5. E

Petit mal epilepsy describes transient 'absences' or blank spells which invariably begin in childhood and virtually never continue beyond adolescence although it may be followed by adult epilepsy. The EEG shows typical spike and wave complexes at 3/second and sodium valproate is the drug of first choice.

6. ABD

Lumbar puncture is often useful in establishing the diagnosis of multiple sclerosis. Lymphocytosis and increased protein may be present. Immunoelectrophoresis is particularly helpful and may show raised IgG and oligoclonal bands. A negative VDRL is helpful in excluding neurosyphilis.

7. **In Friedreich's ataxia**
   A Clinical manifestations are unusual before the age of 40
   B Dorsal column loss occurs
   C Pyramidal weakness occurs
   D Optic atrophy may develop
   E Death may occur from heart failure

8. **In Huntington's chorea**
   A Inheritance is autosomal recessive
   B Raised levels of gamma amino butyric acid (GABA) are found in the brain
   C The onset of symptoms usually occurs in adolescence
   D The chorea may respond to tetrabenazine
   E Life expectancy is normal

7. BCDE

In Friedreich's ataxia, degeneration in the dorsal and lateral columns, spinocerebellar tracts, and sometimes optic nerves, leads to clinical manifestations in the early teens. Arrythmias and cardiac failure are common and due to cardiomyopathy.

8. D

Huntington's chorea is inherited as an autosomal dominant and usually presents between 30 and 45. A loss of neurons which normally contain GABA has been demonstrated in the corpus striatum. These neurons have an inhibitory effect on dopaminergic neurons in the substantia nigra. Hence drugs which deplete dopamine stores such as tetrabenazine may have a beneficial effect. The disease usually progresses to death within 10 to 15 years.

9. **In myotonia dystrophica**
    A Ovarian atrophy occurs
    B IQ is usually normal
    C Visual disturbance may result from optic atrophy
    D Myotonia may be absent
    E Muscle wasting occurs

10. **In Duchenne muscular dystrophy**
    A CPK is elevated at birth
    B CPK may be elevated in female carriers
    C Life expectancy is normal
    D Muscle wasting is an early sign
    E Presentation usually occurs in early teens

9. ADE

Myotonia dystrophica is inherited as an autosomal dominant but expression is very variable. Classical features include frontal balding, ptosis, muscle wasting, mental deficiency, cataracts and gonadal atrophy. Clinical myotonia may be absent but detectable on EMG.

10. AB

Duchenne muscular dystrophy is a sex linked recessive disorder which usually presents when the child begins to walk. An elevated CPK has been found in cord blood and CPK may be elevated in female carriers. Muscle hypertrophy is common (pseudo-hypertrophy). Death usually occurs from respiratory failure in early teens.

11. The following may be useful in the treatment of a depressive illness
   A Amitriptyline
   B Reserpine
   C Phenelzine
   D α methyl dopa
   E Mianserin

12. Alzheimer's disease is characterized by
   A Loss of memory for recent more than past events
   B Emotional lability
   C Paranoid delusions
   D Auditory hallucinations
   E Preservation of insight

11. ACE

The usefulness of tricyclic and tetracyclic antidepressants (such as amitriptyline and mianserin) and monoamine oxidase inhibitors (such as phenelzine) in the treatment of depression is thought to relate to their effects on cerebral amines. Tricyclic antidepressants prevent the re-uptake of released noradrenaline, and monoamine oxidase inhibitors prevent the breakdown of both seretonin and catecholamines. Reserpine and α methyl dopa may both produce depression when used in the treatment of hypertension.

12. AC

Alzheimer's disease is the commonest form of dementia and results in a global loss of cognitive function. The onset is usually insidious and loss of short-term memory is one of the earliest features. Insight is lost early and the course is steadily progressive with the development of abnormal behaviour, failure to learn, reduction in self care, incontinence, blunting of emotions and paranoia.

13. **Schizophrenia**
   A   Usually presents in early adult life
   B   May be familial
   C   May be precipitated by a physical illness
   D   Is often associated with visual hallucinations
   E   Is often associated with a lack of contact with reality

14. **Korsakoff's syndrome**
   A   Usually occurs in alcoholics
   B   Is associated with loss of short-term memory
   C   Is associated with confabulation
   D   May respond to injections of vitamin B_{12}
   E   Is due to a lesion in the frontal lobes

13. ABCE
Schizophrenia is characterized by a number of symptoms, not all of which are present in every case. The main features include disturbance of thought, flattening of affect and withdrawal from reality. Hallucinations are usually auditory and rarely visual. 75% of cases present between 15 and 30 years of age and the onset is usually insidious although a physical illness may act as a precipitating factor. There is good evidence for a familial factor.

14. ABC
Korsakoff's syndrome results from damage to the limbic system and is usually due to thiamine deficiency associated with alcoholism. There is a loss of short-term memory, although immediate memory as tested by immediate recall of a sequence of numbers, is preserved. Confabulation is a common but not invariable feature. Improvement may follow treatment with large doses of intravenous thiamine.

15. Systemic lupus erythematosus (SLE)
A Is commonest in young men
B Rarely causes arthritis
C Is associated with a rash which usually responds to treatment with u.v. light
D May be exacerbated by infection
E Is usually associated with a leucocytosis

16. The following drugs may be useful in the treatment of SLE
A Chloroquine
B Phenytoin
C Salicylates
D Chlorpromazine
E Prednisolone

17. The following laboratory findings would support a diagnosis of polyarteritis nodosa
A Leucopenia
B Eosinophilia
C Positive hepatitis B surface antigen
D Raised ESR
E Weakly positive ANF

18. The following findings would be compatible with a diagnosis of dermatomyositis
A Proximal muscle wasting
B Facial telangiectasia
C Normal CPK
D Normal muscle biopsy
E Spontaneous fibrillation on electromyography

15. D
SLE usually presents in young women. It may be exacerbated by sunlight and infection. Articular problems are one of the commonest manifestations. Leucopenia occurs in two thirds of patients and may be useful in distinguishing the condition from other vasculitides.

16. A C E
SLE usually responds favourably to steroids but arthralgia and arthritis may respond to salicylates alone, and chloroquine may be particularly useful in the management of cutaneous or joint manifestations. Phenytoin and chlorpromazine have both been implicated in the development of drug-induced SLE.

17. B C D E
There is no diagnostic laboratory test for polyarteritis nodosa but the ESR is usually raised and ANF may be present, usually in low titre. The peripheral blood film characteristically shows anaemia, leucocytosis and eosinophilia. There is a recognized association between the presence of hepatitis B surface antigen and the development of polyarteritis nodosa.

18. A B C D E
Dermatomyositis is characterized by proximal muscle weakness, which may progress to muscle wasting and fibrosis, and a telangiectatic rash predominantly affecting the face and trunk. Muscle involvement tends to be patchy and muscle biopsy may therefore be normal. Active degeneration of muscle results in spontaneous fibrillation on electromyography. The degree of active muscle destruction is reflected by the muscle enzymes (such as CPK) which may be normal at times.

19. **In children with juvenile rheumatoid arthritis (Still's disease)**
    A Skin rash and fever are common
    B Joint involvement is usually symmetrical
    C Subcutaneous nodules are common
    D Rheumatoid factor is often absent
    E Iritis is unlikely if ANF is present in plasma

20. **The following occur in Felty's syndrome**
    A Positive rheumatoid factor
    B Positive ANF
    C Leucocytosis
    D Leg ulcers
    E Remission of arthritis following splenectomy

21. **In patients with ankylosing spondylitis**
    A Rheumatoid factor is usually present
    B Fibrosing alveolitis may develop
    C Arthritis may affect peripheral joints
    D Blindness may occur
    E Renal failure may develop

22. **Arthritis in Reiter's syndrome**
    A May follow an episode of bacillary dysentry
    B Is usually symmetrical affecting small joints
    C Usually remits spontaneously
    D Rarely progresses to permanent joint deformity
    E Is commoner in patients with HLA B27

19. AD

Systemic features such as lymphadenopathy, splenomegaly, rash and fever are common in juvenile rheumatoid arthritis. The pattern of joint involvement is variable and may be monoarticular. Tests for rheumatoid factor are usually negative and subcutaneous nodules are rare. A strong association has been found between the presence of ANF and the development of iritis.

20. ABD

In Felty's syndrome (rheumatoid arthritis, splenomegaly and neutropenia), the rheumatoid factor is usually strongly positive and ANF is often present. Leg ulceration may result from cutaneous vasculitis. Splenectomy may improve haematological abnormalities but does not affect the underlying rheumatoid process.

21. BCDE

Patients with ankylosing spondylitis have an increased incidence of iritis, aortitis, fibrosing alveolitis and ulcerative colitis. Rheumatoid factor is usually absent. Peripheral joints are involved in 25% of patients. Renal failure may result from amyloid, analgesic nephropathy, or, in patients treated with radiotherapy, radiation nephritis.

22. ACE

In the UK, Reiter's syndrome usually follows an episode of sexually transmitted non-specific urethritis but may also follow bacillary dysentry. The arthritis is usually asymmetrical affecting large joints. Attacks tend to remit spontaneously but recurrence with progression to permanent deformity is not uncommon. HLA B27 is present in 75% of cases.

23. The following are recognized findings in Graves' disease

A Unilateral exophthalmos

B Persistence of exophthalmos following treatment of thyroid disease

C Papilloedema

D Diplopia

E Eye signs in the absence of hyperthyroidism

24. Medullary (C-cell) carcinoma of the thyroid

A May secrete calcitonin

B Usually causes hypocalcaemia

C Should be treated surgically

D May be treated with radioactive iodine

E Has an association with phaeochromocytoma

25. Acromegaly

A Is usually caused by a basophil pituitary adenoma

B May be caused by a chromophobe pituitary adenoma

C Is associated with diabetes

D Is associated with an increased incidence of renal stones

E May respond to treatment with bromocriptine

23. ABCDE

Exophthalmos may be asymmetrical in Graves' disease and often persists despite treatment of the thyroid disease. It is due to swelling of the orbital contents. In severe cases pressure on the optic nerve, resulting in papilloedema and ultimately blindness, may require surgical decompression. Diplopia may result from ophthalmoplegia. In ophthalmic Graves' disease, eye signs occur in the absence of hyperthyroidism.

24. ACE

Although medullary (C-cell) carcinoma may secrete calcitonin (in addition to ACTH and serotonin), hypocalcaemia is rare. The medullary C-cells do not take up iodine and thus surgery is the treatment of choice. It may occur as part of the multiple endocrine adenomatosis (MEA) syndrome together with phaeochromocytoma and parathyroid adenoma.

25. BCDE

Basophil adenomas usually secrete ACTH, growth hormone usually being secreted by acidophil or, more rarely, chromophobe adenomas. Growth hormone antagonizes the action of insulin and diabetes may result. Hypercalcaemia and hypercalciuria occur and may cause renal stones. Growth hormone release is usually stimulated by dopamine but is paradoxically inhibited by the dopamine agonist bromocriptine in acromegaly.

26. **The following may be found in Addison's disease**
    A   Raised blood urea
    B   Raised plasma sodium
    C   Low plasma chloride
    D   Low plasma potassium
    E   Low blood glucose

27. **Metyrapone**
    A   Inhibits 11-β hydroxylation of corticosteroids in the adrenal gland
    B   Reduces plasma cortisol in normal people
    C   Reduces urinary 17-oxogenic steroid excretion in normal people
    D   Increases urinary 17-oxogenic steroid excretion in patients with ectopic ACTH production
    E   May be useful in the treatment of Cushing's disease

28. **Secretion of prolactin by the anterior pituitary is stimulated by**
    A   L-dopa
    B   Thyrotropin releasing hormone
    C   Pregnancy
    D   Bromocriptine
    E   Chlorpromazine

26. ACE

Blood urea levels may be raised in Addison's disease due to reduced plasma volume and hypotension lowering the glomerular filtration rate. The reduced plasma volume results in a rise in plasma vasopressin and water retention which together with aldosterone deficiency may result in a fall in plasma sodium and chloride levels. Lack of aldosterone may also result in a rise of plasma potassium. Hypoglycaemia may result from the lack of the antagonistic effect of cortisol on insulin.

27. ABE

Metyrapone inhibits $11-\beta$ hydroxylase in the adrenal gland which then produces 11-deoxycortisol instead of cortisol. The fall in cortisol causes a rise in pituitary ACTH production except when this is suppressed by ectopic ACTH or corticosteroid-producing adrenal tumours. In normal people and people with pituitary-dependent Cushing's this rise in ACTH stimulates further production, and hence urinary excretion, of 17-oxogenic steroids

28. BCE

The secretion of prolactin is under inhibitory control by a hormone secreted by the hypothalamus which is probably dopamine. Secretion is therefore inhibited by L-dopa and the dopamine agonist bromocriptine, and stimulated by drugs which block dopamine receptors such as chlorpromazine. Secretion is also stimulated by TRH and during pregnancy.

29. **In a patient with a plasma sodium of 110 mmol/l the following would suggest a diagnosis of inappropriate ADH secretion**
A   Raised blood urea
B   Hypotension
C   Urine osmolality greater than that of plasma
D   Collapsed left lower lobe on chest X-ray
E   Oedema

30. **Phaeochromocytoma**
A   Is derived from chromaffin tissue
B   Usually arises in the adrenal medulla
C   In extramedullary sites usually secretes adrenaline
D   Is usually malignant
E   May be familial

29. CD

With inappropriate ADH secretion water intoxication occurs as a result of excessive tubular reabsorption. Urine osmolality is high and blood urea tends to be low. A raised blood urea and hypotension would suggest sodium depletion. Oedema is unusual. Inappropriate ADH secretion may occur as a result of carcinoma of the bronchus (particularly oat cell) and chest infections.

30. ABE

90% of phaeochromocytomata arise in the adrenal medulla but only 10% are malignant. They stain brown with dichromate, hence their designation chromaffin. The enzyme required for conversion of noradrenaline to adenaline is found only in the adrenal medulla and thus an extramedullary phaeochromocytoma secretes largely noradrenaline. Phaeochromocytoma may be associated with neurofibromatosis and the multiple endocrine adenomatosis syndrome.

31. In patients with diabetic nephropathy
    A   Structural changes in the kidney are usually present at the onset of diabetes
    B   Proteinuria is rare
    C   Progression to renal failure is uncommon
    D   Metformin may be useful in improving diabetic control
    E   Chlorpropramide should be given in reduced dosage

32. Fasting hypoglycaemia may occur in
    A   Alcoholism
    B   Retroperitoneal sarcoma
    C   Mesothelioma
    D   Chlorpropramide therapy
    E   Metformin therapy

33. In the carcinoid syndrome
    A   The primary tumour is usually in the appendix
    B   Urinary secretion of 5-hydroxyindole acetic acid is raised
    C   Facial flushing may be aggravated by alcohol
    D   Diarrhoea may be episodic
    E   Pulmonary stenosis may develop

31. E

Proteinuria is usually the first indication of diabetic nephropathy which is uncommon during the first 10 years of diabetes. Once the nephropathy has developed, progression to renal failure is usually inevitable. Biguanides should not be used because of the risk of lactic acidosis. Chlorpropramide is partially excreted unchanged in the kidney and thus dosage should be reduced in renal impairment.

32. ABCD

In the fasting state the liver maintains a normal glucose by glycogenolysis or, if glycogen stores are depleted by a prolonged fast, gluconeogenesis which is inhibited by alcohol. Pancreatic insulinomas are the commonest insulin-producing tumours but extrapancreatic tumours, such as retroperitoneal fibrosarcomas and mesotheliomas may rarely secrete an insulin-related peptide. Hypoglycaemia is a recognized complication of sulphonylureas, which increase endogenous insulin production, but not of biguanides.

33. BCDE

Carcinoid tumours produce several pharmacologically active substances, including 5-hydroxyindoles, which are normally metabolized in the liver. Gut carcinoids do not therefore produce systemic symptoms unless hepatic metastases, which secrete directly into the systemic circulation, are present. Although carcinoid tumours are commonest in the appendix they rarely metastasize. Attacks are characterized by facial flushing, which may be aggravated by alcohol, diarrhoea and wheezing. Right sided valve lesions may occur.

34. **During an attack of acute intermittent porphyria**
    A   Barbiturates may be useful in controlling symptoms of psychosis
    B   Chlorpromazine should be avoided
    C   Urine contains excess porphobilinogen which causes it to darken on standing
    D   Faecal porphyrins are raised
    E   Hypertension is common

35. **In osteoporosis**
    A   Bone mass is reduced
    B   Bone mineralization is abnormal
    C   Serum calcium is usually low
    D   Serum alkaline phosphatase is usually raised
    E   Prolonged immobilization in bed is often required to heal fractures

36. **In Paget's disease of the bone**
    A   Serum alkaline phosphatase is usually normal
    B   24 hour urinary hydroxyproline levels are raised
    C   Osteolytic lesions occur
    D   Osteosclerotic lesions occur
    E   Bone pain may respond to treatment with calcitonin

34. CDE

Attacks of acute intermittent porphyria may be precipitated by various drugs including barbiturates, sulphonamides and the contraceptive pill. Gastrointestinal manifestations, confusion, psychosis, neuropathy, tachycardia and hypertension occur. Chlorpromazine may help to control symptoms. During an acute attack the urine contains excess porphobilinogen, which darkens on standing due to oxidation, the faeces contain excess porphyrins.

35. A

In osteoporosis, bone mass is reduced but mineralization is normal. Serum calcium, phosphate and alkaline phosphatase are all normal. Prolonged immobilization is a recognized cause of osteoporosis and bed rest following fractures should be minimized.

36. BCDE

In Paget's disease, increased osteoclastic resorption of bone (causing osteolytic lesions) is associated with abnormal new bone formation (causing osteosclerotic lesions). The increased bone turnover is reflected by increased serum alkaline phosphatase and increased 24 hour urinary hydroxyproline excretion. Calcitonin inhibits osteoclastic activity and thus may be useful in treatment.

37. **The following are features of primary hyper-parathyroidism**
    A   A benign parathyroid adenoma is the commonest cause
    B   Peptic ulceration
    C   Corneal calcification
    D   Osteolytic bone lesions
    E   Polyuria

38. **The following drugs may precipitate an attack of gout**
    A   Indomethacin
    B   Thiazide diuretics
    C   Allopurinol
    D   Aspirin
    E   Colchicine

37. ABCDE

90% of cases of primary hyperparathyroidism are due to benign adenomas. Parathyroid hormone induces osteolysis and may produce radiological evidence of generalized osteo-porosis or areas of bone resorption and cysts. Many of the clinical features, including polyuria and corneal calcification are due to the effects of hypercalcaemia. The increased incidence of peptide ulceration may be due to hypercalcaemia stimulating gastrin production.

38. BCD

Diuretics and salicylates in low doses both reduce urinary uric acid excretion. Allopurinol reduces urate production by inhibiting xanthine oxidase production but may precipitate gout in the early stages of treatment, probably due to mobil-ization of uric acid from tophi. Colchicine is particularly effective in relieving acute gout but may produce gastro-intestinal symptoms. Indomethacin may be useful in reducing inflammation.

39. In the nephrotic syndrome
 A Underlying diabetes mellitus is present in about half of all cases
 B Oedema may be absent
 C Proteinuria is usually greater than 5g/24 hours
 D The serum albumin may be normal
 E Proteinuria is usually selective in minimal change glomerulonephritis

40. The following may cause haematuria
 A Renal calculi
 B Cyclophosphamide
 C Urinary tract infection
 D Porphyria
 E Paroxysmal nocturnal haemoglobinuria

41. The following are characteristic of pre-renal uraemia
 A Hypertension
 B Red cell casts in the urine
 C Polyuria
 D Inevitable progression to renal failure
 E Urinary sodium excretion of 100 mmol/1

39. CE

The nephrotic syndrome is defined as the presence of proteinuria, usually in excess of 5 g/24 hours, hypoalbuminaemia and oedema. The commonest cause is glomerulonephritis (about 80% of cases). The differential protein excretion is determined by measuring the renal clearance of endogenous IgG (a large molecule) and transferrin (a small molecule). A ratio of these of less than 0.2 indicates selective proteinuria which is characteristic of minimal change glomerulonephritis.

40. ABC

Common causes of haematuria are renal stones, urinary tract infection and urothelial or renal tumours. Metabolites of cyclophosphamide may produce a haemorrhagic cystitis. Microscopic identification of red cells in the urine distinguishes haematuria from haemoglobinuria (as in paroxysmal nocturnal haemoglobinuria) or other causes of red urine (such as porphobilinogen).

41. None

In pre-renal uraemia, renal underperfusion usually results from prolonged hypotension. The diagnosis implies that renal parenchymal damage has not occurred. Cellular casts are therefore absent and correction of hypovolaemia may prevent renal failure. The kidneys respond physiologically and produce small volumes of urine with a low sodium (less than 10 mmol/l) and high urea content.

42. **Nephrogenic diabetes insipidus may occur in**
A Chronic pyelonephritis
B Analgesic nephropathy
C Craniopharyngioma
D Hypokalaemia
E Hypocalcaemia

43. **In Goodpasture's syndrome**
A Renal damage is mediated by circulating immune complexes
B Anti-glomerular basement membrane antibodies may be detected in plasma
C Men are more frequently affected
D Haemoptysis may occur
E Pulmonary gas transfer may be increased

44. **Urinary tract infection**
A Is commoner in women
B Is usually caused by *E. coli*
C If caused by pseudomonas suggests structural abnormality to the urinary tract
D May be confirmed by finding more than 1000 organisms /ml of urine
E May be asymptomatic

42. ABD
Nephrogenic diabetes insipidus results from an inability of the renal tubes to respond to ADH. Usually there is tubular damage as in chronic pyelonephritis and analgesic nephropathy, but it may also result from hypokalaemia and hypercalcaemia.

43. BCDE
Renal damage in Goodpasture's syndrome is due to anti-glomerular basement membrane antibodies, unlike other forms of glomerulonephritis in which circulating immune complexes are involved. Antibody production may be triggered by occupational exposure to organic chemicals explaining the higher incidence in young men. The basement membrane of lung tissue may also be affected giving rise to pulmonary haemorrhage, which increases pulmonary gas transfer, and haemoptysis.

44. ABCE
The shorter female urethra is thought to predispose women to transperineal infection of urine with bowel organisms. *E. coli* is the commonest pathogen and the presence of other organisms suggests structural abnormality of the urinary tract or instrumentation. Bacteriuria is confirmed by finding more than 100,000 organisms/ml of urine, counts of less than 10,000/ml usually being due to contamination. Infection may be symptom free.

45. Analgesic nephropathy
 A Causes an interstitial nephritis
 B Occurs following ingestion of large amounts of phenacetin
 C Is associated with an increased incidence of urothelial tumours
 D Rarely progresses to renal failure
 E May improve following cessation of analgesic abuse

46. In adult polycystic disease
 A Inheritance is autosomal recessive
 B Haematuria is common
 C Nephrotic syndrome is common
 D Ultrasound may be useful in diagnosis
 E Cysts may also be present in the liver

45. ABCE
Chronic ingestion of analgesics, particularly phenacetin, may cause interstitial nephritis and necrosis of renal papillae. Discontinuation of analgesics often results in stabilization or improvement in renal function whereas continued consumption leads to progressive renal damage. About 10% of patients develop transitional cell tumours of the renal pelvis and ureter.

46. BDE
Adult polycystic disease is inherited as an autosomal dominant. Cysts may also be present in the liver and can usually be detected by ultrasound. Haematuria due to haemorrhage into cysts or infection is common. Proteinuria may occur but is rarely severe enough to be clinically significant.

47. Hepatitis A
   A   Is a DNA virus
   B   Has an incubation period of 3 to 6 months
   C   Is transmitted by the faecal-oral route
   D   Is usually diagnosed by detecting the virus in urine
   E   May progress to chronic liver disease

48. Chronic active hepatitis
   A   May follow hepatitis B infection
   B   Is characterized histologically by piecemeal necrosis
       and rosette formation in liver lobules
   C   Is associated with a markedly raised serum IgM
   D   Is associated with the presence of serum antibodies
       against smooth muscle
   E   Rarely progresses to cirrhosis

49. Alcoholic cirrhosis
   A   Is usually micronodular
   B   Is characterized histologically by fibrosis with
       regeneration of liver cells
   C   May be reversible following abstinence from alcohol
   D   Predisposes to the development of hepatocellular
       carcinoma
   E   Causes hepatomegaly only when advanced

47. C

Hepatitis A is a picornavirus which has an incubation period of 2 to 6 weeks and is transmitted by the faecal-oral route. Although the virus may be found in blood and urine during the early stages of infection, it is more readily demonstrated in faeces. The diagnosis is usually made by demonstrating IgM antibodies to hepatitis A in serum. Chronic liver disease does not develop in hepatitis A.

48. ABD

In chronic active hepatitis the aetiology is often unknown (probably an autoimmune process) or there may be a preceeding history of viral hepatitis (B or non-A-non-B). Histologically there is piecemeal necrosis within the liver lobules with areas of fibrosis isolating liver cells in the form of rosettes. Serum IgG is usually very high and smooth muscle antibodies are found in about 60% of cases. Progression to cirrhosis is common.

49. ABD

Cirrhosis is a pathological diagnosis implying both hepatic fibrosis and nodular regeneration of liver cells. In alcoholism it is usually micronodular and is irreversible once established. Although hepatomegaly is a common early feature progressive fibrosis often causes shrinkage of the liver. Progression to hepatocellular carcinoma may occur.

50. The following are features of primary biliary cirrhosis
A   Pruritus
B   Pigmentation
C   Clubbing
D   Raised serum IgE
E   Anti-mitochondrial antibodies

51. In portal hypertension
A   The portal pressure is usually greater than 15 mmHg
B   An umbilical venous hum may be present
C   Gastric varices may occur
D   Thrombocytopenia may occur
E   Schistosoma haematobium may be important aetiologically

52. In ascites due to chronic liver disease
A   The total protein content of ascitic fluid is usually less than 25 g/l
B   Therapeutic aspiration is usually necessary
C   A low salt diet may be useful in management
D   Spironolactone should be avoided
E   Treatment with diuretics may precipitate encephalopathy

50. ABCE
Primary biliary cirrhosis is a disease predominantly of middle aged women in which a micronodular cirrhosis results from chronic biliary obstruction at the level of biliary ductules. Pruritus is often the presenting feature and jaundice, pigmentation, xanthomas, hepatosplenomegaly and clubbing are common. Serum IgM is usually raised and anti-mitochondrial antibodies are present in over 90% of patients.

51. ABCD
The normal portal pressure is 5–10 mmHg and clinical features of portal hypertension usually become apparent with pressures greater than 15 mmHg. The development of collateral channels between the portal and systemic circulation may result in varices in the oesophagus and cardia of the stomach and recanalization of the umbilical vein. Splenomegaly may develop and lead to thrombocytopenia. Although hepatic schistosomiasis (usually with *S. mansoni*) may be aetiologically important, schistosoma haematobium predominantly infects the urinary tract.

52. ACE
Ascites in chronic liver disease is usually a transudate with a protein content less than 25 g/l. Therapeutic aspiration is usually unhelpful as fluid tends to re-accumulate and excessive protein loss may occur. Treatment should usually be with a low salt diet and diuretics, incorporating a potassium-sparing diuretic to avoid hypokalaemia. Diuretic therapy may however precipitate encephalopathy due to volume depletion or electrolyte imbalance.

53. Haemochromatosis
A   Is inherited as a sex-linked condition
B   Results in pigmentation due to deposition of melanin in the skin
C   May present with diabetes
D   Is associated with the development of cardiac failure
E   Should be treated with desferrioxamine

54. The following are features of Wilson's disease
A   Raised serum caeruloplasmin
B   Raised 24 hour urinary copper excretion
C   Amino-aciduria
D   Glycosuria
E   Kayser–Fleischer rings

53. BCD
Haemochromatosis is an autosomally inherited error of metabolism resulting in excess iron absorption, but clinical features are less common in women presumably due to continual iron losses from menstruation. Homozygotes are more markedly affected than heterozygotes. Iron deposition occurs in various organs including liver, heart, pancreas and endocrine glands. Skin pigmentation is common, resulting largely from deposition of melanin rather than iron. Excess iron is best removed by regular venesection.

54. BCDE
The basic genetic defect in Wilson's disease is unknown but impaired biliary excretion of copper and impaired production of caeruloplasmin, a glycoprotein which carries copper in the serum, result in excess deposition of copper in the liver, brain, kidney (resulting in defects of tubular absorption) and eye (as Kayser–Fleischer rings).

55. The following findings on a barium meal would suggest that a gastric ulcer was benign
A Ulcer sited on the greater curve
B Raised edges to the ulcer
C Smooth mucosal folds radiating towards the base of the ulcer
D Evidence of previous partial gastrectomy
E Loss of peristalsis around the ulcer

56. In the Zollinger–Ellison syndrome
A A gastrin-producing adenoma is usually present in the pancreas
B The tumour is usually malignant
C Gastric acid secretion increases dramatically in response to pentagastrin
D Jejunal ulceration may occur
E Diarrhoea may be a presenting feature

57. In acute gastrointestinal bleeding
A The commonest site of bleeding is a gastric ulcer
B Presentation may be with fresh rectal bleeding
C Serum creatinine may be raised due to absorption of protein from the gut
D Fibre optic endoscopy should be avoided if possible
E The prognosis is worse in the elderly

55. C

Malignant gastric ulcers are commoner on the greater curve although they may occur at other sites. They are often irregular in outline with raised rolled margins and irregularity or loss of the adjacent mucosal folds. Reduction or absence of peristalsis in the area of the ulcer suggests underlying infiltration. Carcinoma of the stomach is commoner in gastric remnants following partial gastrectomy.

56. ADE

In the Zollinger–Ellison syndrome a gastrin-producing adenoma is usually found in the body or tail of the pancreas although it may occur in the spleen, stomach or duodenum. Gastric acid secretion is persistently raised and rises little further following pentagastrin. Recurrent peptic ulceration which may extend into the jejunum is a characteristic feature and diarrhoea is not uncommon. About one third of tumours become malignant.

57. BE

Acute upper gastrointestinal bleeding most commonly arises from duodenal ulceration and if massive may present with fresh rectal bleeding. Protein absorption from the gut may result in a rise in blood urea but a raised creatinine indicates renal impairment as a result of hypovolaemia or pre-existing renal failure. If available fibre optic endoscopy should be performed as soon as the patient is stable to identify the source of bleeding. The prognosis is worse in the elderly and has led to a tendency to operate earlier in such patients.

58. **In ulcerative colitis**
A   There is always rectal involvement
B   Oral ulceration may occur
C   Colonic carcinoma is usually an early complication
D   The incidence of cholangiocarcinoma is increased
E   The incidence of ankylosing spondylitis is increased

59. **The following are recognized complications of Crohn's disease**
A   Erythema nodosum
B   Pyoderma gangrenosum
C   Renal calculi
D   Colonic carcinoma
E   Amyloid

60. **Patients with coeliac disease (gluten-sensitive enteropathy)**
A   May present in adult life
B   Should avoid foods containing maize
C   May eat rye bread
D   Can usually return to a normal diet once remission has been induced
E   Have an increased incidence of intestinal lymphoma

58. ABDE

Ulcerative colitis is a distal disease in which the rectum is always involved with variable extension proximally. Although inflammation is limited to the large bowel, aphthous ulceration may occur in the mouth. The risk of developing colonic carcinoma increases with time. Rarely, patients may develop carcinoma of the bile duct. The incidence of ankylosing spondylitis is increased and patients who suffer from both tend to have HLA B27.

59. ABCDE

Erythema nodosum and pyoderma gangrenosum are the commonest cutaneous manifestations of Crohn's disease. There is an increased incidence of renal stones, particularly urate and oxalate, which may relate to episodes of dehydration, urinary infection, ureteric obstruction or reduced urinary pH. There is a recognized increase in colonic carcinoma in Crohn's colitis. Amyloid may occur in the bowel or systemically and may regress following resection of affected bowel.

60. AE

Coeliac disease may present in infancy or childhood, usually with gastrointestinal symptoms or failure to thrive, or adulthood when symptoms are often non-specific. Wheat, rye, barley and malt should be avoided but maize, rice and oats are harmless. Treatment needs to be lifelong as relapse follows reintroduction of gluten into the diet. Coeliac disease is associated with an increased incidence of gastrointestinal malignancy, particularly lymphoma.

61. **After ingestion of 5 g of D-xylose**
   A Xylose is predominantly absorbed in the duodenum
   B More than 1 g is usually excreted in the urine in the following 5 hours
   C Urinary excretion may be reduced in coeliac disease
   D Urinary excretion may be reduced in chronic pancreatitis
   E Urinary excretion may be reduced in chronic pyelonephritis

62. **Carcinoma of the pancreas**
   A Is usually an adenocarcinoma
   B Most commonly occurs in the tail of the pancreas
   C Is unlikely if there is dilatation of the gallbladder
   D May present with fluctuating jaundice
   E May present with superficial venous thrombosis

61. BCE

Xylose is mainly absorbed in the jejunum and more than 20% (1 g) of a 25 g oral load is normally excreted in the urine in the 5 hours after ingestion. Urinary excretion is reduced in intestinal, but not pancreatic, malabsorption and renal disease.

62. ADE

Pancreatic carcinoma is most commonly an adenocarcinoma of ductal cell origin and about 75% occur in the head. Progressive obstructive jaundice and in some cases dilatation of the gallbladder result from biliary obstruction. An ampullary carcinoma may rarely lead to intermittent jaundice. Recurrent superficial venous thromboses (thrombophlebitis migrans) are not uncommon and may be the presenting feature.

63. Cystic fibrosis
- **A** Is commoner in males
- **B** May be diagnosed if the sweat sodium concentration is less than 20 mmol/l
- **C** Is associated with sterility in males
- **D** May cause steatorrhoea
- **E** Is associated with a normal life expectancy

64. In a patient with asthma the following values would be reduced
- **A** Forced expiratory volume in 1 second (FEV_1)
- **B** Forced vital capacity (FVC)
- **C** FEV_1/FVC ratio
- **D** Peak expiratory flow rate
- **E** Functional residual capacity

65. Respiratory syncytial virus
- **A** Is the principal cause of bronchiolitis in infancy
- **B** Induces syncytial formation in tissue culture
- **C** Causes winter epidemics
- **D** Is unlikely to be the cause of a respiratory infection if a skin rash is present
- **E** Responds to tetracycline

66. Lung abscess formation typically complicates pneumonia due to
- **A** *Staphylococcus aureus*
- **B** *Haemophilus influenzae*
- **C** *Klebsiella pneumoniae*
- **D** *Mycoplasma pneumoniae*
- **E** Respiratory syncytial virus

63. CD

Cystic fibrosis is an autosomal recessive disorder affecting exocrine glands in which the principal abnormalities are increased viscosity of secreted mucus and a raised sodium concentration in the sweat (more than 70 mmol/l). Recurrent respiratory infections and pancreatic insufficiency predominate but the salivary glands, sinuses, bile ducts and seminiferous tubules are also affected. The prognosis has improved recently with improved treatment of respiratory problems with physiotherapy and antibiotics, and increasing numbers of sufferers are surviving into adult life.

64. ABCD

Airways obstruction in asthma results in a reduction in FEV_1, vital capacity, FEV_1/FVC ratio and peak expiratory flow rate. Overinflation of the chest may lead to an increase in functional residual capacity and residual volume.

65. ABC

Respiratory syncytial virus is a common cause of bronchiolitis and bronchopneumonia in infancy. It may be identified by immunofluorescence techniques from nasopharyngeal secretions or tracheal aspirates and induces syncytial formation in tissue culture. Infection generally occurs in winter epidemics and may be associated with an erythematous rash. It is not responsive to antibiotics.

66. AC

Necrosis within a consolidated area of pneumonia may result in cavitation and abscess formation. This occurs frequently in staphylococcal and klebsiella pneumonia and is an occasional complication of pneumococcal pneumonia.

67. **Bronchial adenoma**
    A   Is usually a carcinoid tumour
    B   Is always benign
    C   Can rarely be visualized by bronchoscopy
    D   May present with recurrent pneumonia
    E   May present with haemoptysis

68. **Isoniazid**
    A   Is a bactericidal anti-tuberculous agent
    B   Is acetylated to an active compound in the liver
    C   Does not cross the blood-brain barrier
    D   May cause a peripheral neuropathy
    E   Colours the urine orange

69. **Farmer's lung**
    A   Is an example of a type I hypersensitivity reaction
    B   Is characterized by cough and dyspnoea immediately following exposure to mouldy hay
    C   Is associated with a restrictive ventilatory defect
    D   Is associated with a reduced transfer factor
    E   May progress to irreversible pulmonary fibrosis

70. **In cryptogenic fibrosing alveolitis**
    A   Clubbing rarely occurs
    B   The incidence of bronchial carcinoma is increased
    C   Cyanosis may occur after exercise
    D   Arterial P_{CO_2} may be reduced
    E   There is usually a raised FEV_1/FVC ratio

67. ADE

90% of bronchial adenomata are carcinoid tumours, the majority of the remainder being cylindromata. They tend to occur in the large bronchi and can usually be visualized by bronchoscopy. Haemoptysis is a common presenting feature and bronchial obstruction may lead to recurrent infections. Although the majority are benign, distant metastases occur in about 10% of cases.

68. AD

Isoniazid is a bactericidal anti-tuberculous agent which readily enters the CSF and is thus particularly useful in the treatment of tuberculous meningitis. It is inactivated by acetylation. It interferes with pyridoxine metabolism and may induce pyridoxine deficiency resulting in a peripheral neuropathy. Rifampicin colours the urine orange.

69. CDE

In farmer's lung a type III (precipitin-mediated) hypersensitivity reaction to thermophilic actinomycetes results in alveolar and interstitial inflammation 1 to 6 hours after exposure to mouldy hay. A restrictive ventilatory defect and reduced transfer factor are characteristic. Changes are reversible in the early stages if exposure is avoided but repeated exposure may lead to irreversible pulmonary fibrosis.

70. BCDE

In cryptogenic fibrosing alveolitis progressive pulmonary fibrosis causes a restrictive defect on spirometry. A normal arterial Po_2 may be maintained by hyperventilation causing a reduced Pco_2 but the Po_2 falls on exercise. Clubbing occurs in two thirds of cases and the incidence of bronchial carcinoma is increased.

71. **The following are features of Dressler's post myocardial infarction syndrome**
   A Onset within the first week following myocardial infarction
   B Pericarditis
   C Pleurisy
   D Fever
   E Antibodies to smooth muscle

72. **Rheumatic fever**
   A Most commonly occurs in young adults
   B Follows a group B streptococcal infection
   C May cause a myocarditis
   D May cause painful subcutaneous nodules
   E Rarely recurs

73. **The ductus arteriosus**
   A Connects the pulmonary artery to the ascending aorta
   B Usually closes prior to birth
   C Fibroses to form the ligamentum arteriosum
   D May undergo delayed closure in premature infants
   E If patent may close following administration of indomethacin

71. BCD

Dressler's post myocardial infarction syndrome usually occurs several weeks after infarction and is characterized by fever, pericarditis and pleurisy. It is thought to be an auto-immune reaction to damaged heart muscle, and antibodies to cardiac muscle have been detected in some cases.

72. C

Rheumatic fever follows a group A β haemolytic strepto-coccal infection and usually occurs between the ages of 5 and 15. Endocarditis is usually recognized by the development of heart murmurs but myocarditis and pericarditis are also common. Polyarthritis, painless subcutaneous nodules, erythema marginatum and chorea are other clinical features. Recurrence is not uncommon and prophylaxis against further streptococcal infections with penicillin is indicated in affected patients.

73. CDE

The ductus arteriosus connects the left pulmonary artery to the descending aorta. Its closure during the first few days of life is thought to relate to several factors including reduced pulmonary vascular resistance, a rise in the oxygen tension of blood perfusing the duct and a fall in circulating prosta-glandins. Closure may be delayed in premature infants and indomethacin, a prostaglandin synthetase inhibitor, may be helpful in inducing closure in such cases.

74. **Fallot's tetralogy is associated with**
   A Cyanosis
   B Anaemia
   C Left to right shunting
   D Squatting
   E Pulmonary plethora on chest X-ray

75. **The following are features of Eisenmenger's syndrome**
   A Right to left shunt
   B Presentation at birth
   C Cyanosis
   D Haemoptysis
   E Clubbing

76. **In hypertrophic cardiomyopathy**
   A There may be a familial incidence
   B A slow rising pulse is characteristic
   C Atrial fibrillation should be treated with digoxin
   D Angina should be treated with GTN
   E β blockers may improve symptoms

74. AD

Fallot's tetralogy is characterized by a ventricular septal defect, right ventricular outflow obstruction, right ventricular hypertrophy and overriding of the interventricular septum by the aorta. The right ventricular outflow obstruction results in right to left shunting across the ventricular septal defect reducing pulmonary blood flow (resulting in oligaemic lung fields on chest X-ray) and causing arterial hypoxaemia (resulting in cyanosis and polycythaemia). Squatting compresses the abdominal aorta increasing the systemic arterial resistance and reducing the left to right shunt.

75. ACDE

Eisenmenger originally described a patient with a ventricular septal defect in whom the development of pulmonary hypertension resulted in a right to left shunt. The term Eisenmenger's syndrome has been extended to include any connection between the two sides of the heart (at atrial, ventricular or aorto-pulmonary level) in which the pulmonary vascular resistance becomes greater than the systemic vascular resistance with a resultant right to left shunt. The clinical features, which usually develop during adolescence or early adult life, are those of pulmonary hypertension with cyanosis.

76. AE

Outflow obstruction occurs in hypertrophic cardiomyopathy due to ventricular muscle hypertrophy giving rise to a characteristic steep rising jerky pulse. Stimulating myocardial contraction (with digoxin) or reducing afterload (with GTN) exacerbate the obstruction by reducing left ventricular volume. Verapamil and β blockers may help to reduce the obstruction.

82

77. **Right bundle branch block**
    A   May be diagnosed provided that the QRS complex is greater than 0.1 seconds
    B   May occur following pulmonary embolism
    C   May occur transiently during pneumonia
    D   May occur in association with left axis deviation
    E   Is always pathological

78. **In the Wolff–Parkinson–White syndrome**
    A   The PR interval is prolonged
    B   The QRS complex is widened
    C   Recurrent ventricular tachycardia is characteristic
    D   Paroxysmal atrial fibrillation occurs
    E   Digoxin is the treatment of choice

77. BCD

Bundle branch block may be diagnosed if the QRS complex is greater than 0.12 seconds. Right bundle branch block tends to occur in conditions causing right heart strain but need not be pathological. It is usually associated with right axis deviation and the finding of left axis deviation suggests additional left anterior hemi-block.

78. BD

In the Wolff–Parkinson–White syndrome an accessory conduction pathway bypasses the atrio-ventricular node. Early ventricular activation through the bypass tract shortens the PR interval and produces a delta wave at the start of the QRS complex, whilst normal activation through the AV node gives rise to the remainder of the QRS complex. The normal and abnormal conduction pathways form a re-entry circuit facilitating the occurrence of supraventricular tachycardias. Digoxin shortens the refractory period of the bypass tract and if given for atrial fibrillation may increase the ventricular rate and lead to ventricular fibrillation.

79. In psoriasis

    A   Epidermal proliferation is reduced
    B   Extensor surfaces are commonly affected
    C   The scalp is rarely involved
    D   Oral lesions are common
    E   Lesions are aggravated by sunlight

80. The following are features of lichen planus

    A   Wickham's striae
    B   Koebner's phenomenon
    C   Mucosal lesions
    D   Bullous lesions
    E   Nail involvement

81. Atopic eczema

    A   Usually has an onset around puberty
    B   Is often familial
    C   Is associated with asthma
    D   Causes a vesicular rash
    E   Is non-irritant

82. The following may be useful in the treatment of acne vulgaris

    A   u.v. light
    B   Topical corticosteroids
    C   Benzoyl peroxide
    D   Oxytetracycline
    E   Prednisolone

79. B

In psoriasis, increased epidermal proliferation results in the development of well defined, scaly papular lesions. Extensor surfaces and the scalp are most commonly affected although any area of skin may be involved. The oral mucosa is rarely affected. Lesions are often improved by sunlight, and u.v.A light in combination with psoralens (Pu.v.A) is an effective treatment.

80. ABCDE

Lichen planus is characterized by irritating purple, shiny, polygonal papules with fine white lines (Wickham's striae) passing through them. They often occur at sites of injury (Koebner's phenomenon). Lesions of the buccal mucosa and nails are common and may occur in the absence of other skin lesions. Vesicles and bullous lesions may occur, in which case the condition is described as lichen planus bullosus.

81. BCD

Atopy denotes a familial tendency to develop allergic reactions and in addition to eczema there may be a history of hay fever or asthma. Atopic eczema usually presents in infancy giving rise to an irritant vesicular rash which predominantly affects the flexures. The tendency is for spontaneous improvement with the rash in most cases disappearing before puberty.

82. ACD

u.v. light is often beneficial in acne and topical benzoyl peroxide may be effective through both its antiseptic and keratolytic effects. Oral tetracyclines reduce free fatty acid concentration in sebum and inhibit neutrophil chemotaxis in addition to their antibacterial effect and are often effective if topical measures have failed. Oral and topical corticosteroids may both exacerbate acne.

83. Rosacea

A Occurs most commonly during adolescence
B Usually affects the face
C May progress to rhinophyma
D May cause corneal ulceration
E Usually responds to treatment with u.v. light

84. In herpes zoster

A Pain may precede the development of the rash
B *Varicella zoster* virus may be identified in vesicular fluid
C The rash is often bilateral
D Motor nerves may be involved
E An underlying immunoproliferative disorder is usually present

85. Dermatitis herpetiformis

A Causes a non-irritant vesicular rash
B Is associated with HLA B27
C May respond to gluten-free diet
D May respond to treatment with dapsone
E May remit spontaneously

86. Pemphigus vulgaris

A Is associated with IgG deposition in basement membrane on skin biopsy
B May cause widespread skin erosions
C Is associated with a positive Nikolski sign
D Rarely causes oral lesions
E Has a good prognosis

83. BCD

Rosacea usually occurs in middle age giving rise to an erythematous facial rash with papules, pustules and telangiectasia. It is often exacerbated by sunlight and may result in disfiguring hypertrophy of the nose (rhinophyma). An associated conjunctivitis is not uncommon, and keratitis and corneal ulceration may occur in severe cases.

84. ABD

Herpes zoster is due to a reactivation of *Varicella zoster* virus acquired during previous chickenpox infection. Although the incidence is increased in patients with underlying immunological suppression, no cause is apparent in the majority of patients. The characteristic rash is usually preceded by several days of pain. It is confined to one or more dermatomes and is very rarely bilateral. Motor involvement may occur, the facial and ocular nerves being most commonly affected.

85. CDE

The rash in dermatitis herpetiformis is usually intensely irritating. The disease is associated with HLA B8 and gluten-sensitive enteropathy, and may respond to a gluten-free diet. Dapsone also improves the skin lesions. Although it tends to become chronic, spontaneous remission may occur.

86. BC

The lesions in pemphigus vulgaris are superficial (IgG deposition occurs in the intercellular region) causing bullae which rupture easily to cause erosions. The superficial skin layers may be moved over the deeper ones (Nikolski's sign). Oral lesions are common and the prognosis is poor, even on treatment with steroids.

87. **In pernicious anaemia**
   A   Serum vitamin B_{12} levels are normal
   B   Parietal cell and intrinsic factor antibodies may be present
   C   Achlorhydria responds to vitamin B_{12} injections
   D   Peripheral neuropathy may improve following B_{12} injections
   E   Anaemia should be corrected by blood transfusions

88. **The following may be found after severe haemolysis**
   A   Haemoglobinuria
   B   Raised plasma unconjugated bilirubin
   C   Raised plasma haptoglobins
   D   Excess urinary urobilinogen
   E   Low serum iron

89. **The following are features of hereditary spherocytosis**
   A   Autosomal recessive inheritance
   B   Increased permeability of the red cell membrane to sodium
   C   Increased osmotic fragility of red cells
   D   Splenomegaly
   E   Spherocytes disappear from the peripheral blood following splenectomy

87. BD

In pernicious anaemia parietal cell atrophy results in achlorhydria and an absence of intrinsic factor which is required for vitamin B_{12} absorption. Both parietal cell and intrinsic factor antibodies may be found. In addition to the anaemia (which is often associated with a reduced platelet and white cell count) neurological problems may occur (including peripheral neuropathy, subacute combined degeneration of the cord and dementia) and may respond to parenteral vitamin B_{12}. Transfusions may precipitate heart failure and should be avoided if possible.

88. ABD

Haemoglobin released following red cell destruction in haemolysis is carried in the plasma by haptoglobins forming a high molecular weight complex which is not filtered by the glomerulus. In severe haemolysis, haptoglobins may become saturated and free haemoglobin appears in the plasma and urine. Haemoglobin is catabolized by reticuloendothelial cells releasing iron, globin and unconjugated bile pigments which are conjugated in the liver and excreted in the stool. Absorption of excess urobilinogen from the intestine may lead to excess excretion of urobilinogen in the urine.

89. BCD

Hereditary spherocytosis is an autosomal dominant condition in which a defect in the red cell membrane renders it abnormally permeable to sodium. Spherocytes are smaller in diameter with a reduced surface area to volume ratio compared to normal red cells. Their capacity to expand is thus reduced resulting in increased osmotic fragility. Spherocytes are destroyed prematurely in the spleen which is invariably enlarged. Splenectomy prevents the premature red cell destruction although the spherocytosis persists.

90. In sickle cell disease
A Sickling can always be detected at birth
B Valine replaces glutamine on the α chain of haemoglobin
C Splenomegaly is invariable
D Reticulocytosis is usually found
E Jaundice is common

91. In paroxysmal nocturnal haemoglobinuria
A Red cells are more prone to haemolysis in acidified serum
B Red cell acetyl cholinesterase is increased
C Red cells are most commonly found in early morning specimens of urine
D Iron deficiency may occur
E There is an increased tendency to intravascular thrombosis

92. Acute lymphoblastic leukaemia
A Usually affects adults
B May present with bruising
C Is associated with lymphadenopathy
D Is associated with a neutrophilia in the peripheral blood
E May be present if lymphoblasts are absent from the peripheral blood

90. DE

In sickle cell disease valine replaces glutamine in the 6th position on the β chain of haemoglobin. Fetal haemoglobin contains only γ and α chains so sickling may not be detectable at birth. A chronic haemolytic anaemia with raised bilirubin, reticulocytosis and splenomegaly occurs but the spleen may eventually become small due to infarction.

91. ADE

In paroxysmal nocturnal haemoglobinuria an acquired defect renders red cells more sensitive to lysis by complement, particularly in an acid environment (the basis of Ham's test). The red cell membrane is abnormal and red cell acetyl cholinesterase is reduced. Haemolysis occurs, particularly during sleep, leading to haemoglobinuria (but not haematuria) on waking which is often severe enough to cause iron deficiency. There is an increased tendency to thrombotic episodes although the mechanism is unknown.

92. BCE

Acute lymphoblastic leukaemia is the commonest form of leukaemia in childhood. Anaemia, bruising due to thrombocytopenia and lymphadenopathy are the common presenting features. The total white cell count may be normal or raised but an absolute neutropenia is common. Lymphoblasts may be absent from the peripheral blood but are always present in the marrow.

93. **In chronic myeloid leukaemia**
   A The total white cell count is often normal
   B Neutrophil alkaline phosphatase is increased
   C The Philadelphia chromosome may be found in red cell precursors
   D There is usually marked splenic enlargement
   E Lymphadenopathy is a common presenting feature

94. **In infectious mononucleosis (glandular fever)**
   A The causal agent is the Epstein–Barr virus
   B Splenomegaly may occur
   C A characteristic rash often follows administration of penicillin
   D The Paul–Bunnell test may be negative during the first week
   E There is usually a neutrophilia

93. CD

In chronic myeloid leukaemia the peripheral white cell count is usually markedly raised with increased numbers of neutrophils, metamyelocytes, promyelocytes and blast cells. The enzyme alkaline phosphatase is usually deficient in neutrophils and the Philadelphia chromosome, an abnormal chromosome 22 in which the long arm is translocated to chromosome 9 is usually found in leucocytes, red cell precursors and megakaryocytes. The spleen, and in later stages the liver, are usually greatly enlarged but lymphadenopathy is uncommon.

94. ABD

Generalized lymphadenopathy, splenomegaly and a macular-papular rash, more common if ampicillin is given for a sore throat, are characteristic features of infectious mononucleosis. The total white cell count is often increased but the majority of cells are atypical mononuclear cells and neutropenia is usual. The Paul–Bunnell test detects the production of a heterophile IgM antibody which agglutinates sheep red cells and is often negative during the first week.

95. **Following methanol poisoning**
    A There is usually a metabolic alkalosis
    B Blindness may occur
    C Abdominal pain occurs
    D Gastric lavage should be avoided
    E Ethanol should be given

96. **In acute iron poisoning**
    A Upper gastrointestinal bleeding occurs
    B Hepatic necrosis may develop within the first 24 hours
    C Encephalopathy may occur
    D Gastric lavage should be performed with desferrioxamine
    E Desferrioxamine should be given parenterally

95. BCE
Methanol is converted by alcohol dehydrogenase to formaldehyde which inhibits tissue respiration, particularly in the retina and also the pancreas. Formaldehyde is further metabolized to formic acid which accumulates to produce a metabolic acidosis. Treatment includes gastric lavage and ethanol which competitively inhibits the metabolism of methanol by alcohol dehydrogenase.

96. ACDE
Upper gastrointestinal irritation (resulting in epigastric pain, vomiting and haematemesis) may occur within several hours of iron ingestion and may be followed by the development of circulatory collapse, acute renal failure, pulmonary oedema and encephalopathy. Recovery may be followed by the development of hepatic necrosis several days later. Desferrioxamine given orally chelates iron in the stomach and intestine but is not absorbed and should therefore also be given i.m. or by slow i.v. infusion.

97. *Plasmodium vivax* malaria
   A   Is also known as malignant tertian malaria
   B   Rarely causes splenomegaly
   C   Should be treated with primaquine to eradicate the
       liver phase
   D   May cause the nephrotic syndrome
   E   In Africa is often chloroquine resistant

98. Typhoid fever
   A   Is caused by a Gram positive coccus
   B   May be spread by animal contact
   C   Usually presents with diarrhoea
   D   Usually causes a polymorphar leucocytosis
   E   Is a notifiable disease

99. Giardiasis
   A   Is a protozoal infection
   B   Predominantly involves the large intestine
   C   May be asymptomatic
   D   May cause malabsorption
   E   Usually responds to treatment with tetracycline

100. Human Immunodeficiency Virus
   A   Is a retrovirus
   B   May be transmitted by social contact
   C   May be isolated from blood of infected individuals
   D   May be isolated from saliva of infected individuals
   E   May give rise to an asymptomatic carrier state

97. C

The fever in *P. vivax* malaria is characteristically tertian but the course is usually benign (malignant tertian refers to *P. falciparum* malaria in which cerebral and renal complications may occur). Splenomegaly is often an early feature and the rare complication of splenic rupture occurs most commonly in *P. vivax* infections. Treatment with primaquine to eradicate the liver phase and prevent relapses is required in *P. vivax* and *P. ovale* malaria. A chronic asymptomatic erythrocytic parasitaemia may develop in *P. malariae* infection leading to the development in some cases of a malarial nephropathy. Chloroquine resistance is a feature of *P. falciparum* malaria.

98. E

Salmonella typhi is a gram negative rod. It is exclusively a human parasite. Constipation is usually present in the first week and leucopenia is typical. Typhoid should be reported to the public health authorities.

99. ACD

Giardiasis is an infection of the upper small intestine caused by the flagellate protozoan *Giardia lamblia*. It may result in the asymptomatic excretion of cysts in the stool or produce diarrhoea and malabsorption. Metronidazole is the treatment of choice.

100. ACDE

The Human Immunodeficiency Virus (HIV) is the causal agent of Acquired Immunodeficiency Syndrome (AIDS). The virus may be found in the blood, semen, tears and saliva of infected individuals and is transmitted by sexual contact or by injection with infected blood or blood products. It can be identified in asymptomatic carriers who may later develop clinical AIDS.

PART THREE

In this section 60 questions are presented in the format used in the MRCP Part I examination. Ideally these questions should be attempted in one sitting of 2½ hours, writing the answers on a separate sheet using a grid as shown:

	A	B	C	D	E
1	...	...	...	...	...
2	...	...	...	...	...
3	...	...	...	...	...

Question should be answered as T (True), F (False) or D (Don't know) and marked on completion of the paper, +1 for a correct answer, −1 for an incorrect answer and 0 for 'don't know'.

1. **In meningococcal meningitis**
   A Gram positive intracellular diplococci are found in the CSF
   B Blood cultures are rarely positive
   C The CSF sugar is usually normal
   D Penicillin is the treatment of choice
   E Prophylactic treatment should be given to close household contacts

2. **Aldosterone**
   A Is secreted by the zona glomerulosa of the adrenal medulla
   B Causes sodium retention
   C Causes potassium retention
   D Secretion is stimulated by angiotensin II
   E Is antagonized by spironolactone

⊕
Pneumo
staptL
Strep

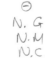
⊖
N. G
N. M
N. C

99

3. **In phenylketonuria**
   A   Inheritance is autosomal recessive
   B   The diagnosis is made by a urine assay on the 6th day of life
   C   Mental retardation may be prevented by a tyrosine free diet
   D   Affected mothers should return to their diet during pregnancy
   E   Eczema is common

4. **The following may be found in normal urine**
   A   Hyaline casts
   B   White cell casts
   C   Red cell casts
   D   Epithelial cells
   E   100 mg protein in a 24 hour collection

5. **In Gilbert's disease**
   A   Inheritance is autosomal dominant
   B   Excess urinary bilirubin is usually detectable
   C   Serum alkaline phosphatase is usually raised
   D   Serum transaminases are normal
   E   Fasting lowers the serum bilirubin

6. **The following findings on colonic biopsy would favour a diagnosis of Crohn's disease rather than ulcerative colitis**
   A   Granuloma formation
   B   Submucosal inflammatory infiltrate
   C   Goblet cell depletion
   D   Crypt abscesses
   E   Superficial ulceration

7. **Oat cell carcinoma of the bronchus**
   A   Is the commonest form of lung cancer
   B   Is associated with cigarette smoking
   C   Rarely metastasizes
   D   May cause hyponatraemia
   E   Is associated with Cushing's syndrome

8. **In a man of 70 with a vertebral collapse the following findings would support a diagnosis of myeloma**
   A   Raised serum calcium
   B   Raised serum alkaline phosphatase
   C   Osteolytic bone lesions
   D   Osteosclerotic bone lesions
   E   40% plasma cells on examination of bone marrow

9. **Ostium secundum atrial septal defect (ASD)**
   A   Is the commonest form of ASD
   B   Usually presents during childhood
   C   Is associated with left axis deviation on ECG
   D   Is associated with wide fixed splitting of the second heart sound
   E   Is a common site of infection in endocarditis

10. **Following subarachnoid haemorrhage**
   A   Glycosuria may occur
   B   ECG changes are common
   C   Recurrence is unusual after the first 48 hours
   D   Diamorphine is the analgesic of choice
   E   Xanthochromia may be absent in the first few hours

101

11. **Rheumatoid factor**
    A   Is a circulating IgM
    B   Has antibody activity against human IgG
    C   Agglutinates sensitized sheep red cells
    D   Is diagnostic of rheumatoid arthritis
    E   If present in high titre in patients with rheumatoid arthritis suggests a poor prognosis

12. **The following are characteristic of the testicular feminization syndrome**
    A   46 XY karyotype
    B   Absent breast enlargement
    C   Primary amenorrhoea
    D   Hirsutism
    E   Increased incidence of gonadal malignancy

13. **Glucagon**
    A   Is a polypeptide
    B   Is secreted by β cells of the Islets of Langerhan
    C   Levels in the plasma are increased during fasting
    D   Inhibits gluconeogenesis
    E   Stimulates glycogenolysis

14. **Hypernephroma (renal cell carcinoma) may present with the following in the absence of metastases**
    A   Anaemia
    B   Polycythaemia
    C   Hypercalcaemia
    D   Abnormal liver function tests
    E   Amyloid

15. Limb girdle (Erb) muscular dystrophy
A   Is transmitted as an autosomal recessive
B   Usually presents in infancy
C   Rarely causes severe disability
D   Is associated with a raised serum CPK
E   Commonly involves the cranial muscles

16. Parietal cells
A   Are found in the antrum of the stomach
B   Produce gastric acid
C   Secrete gastrin
D   Secrete pepsinogens
E   Are found in excess in pernicious anaemia

17. Mesothelioma
A   Only occurs after heavy exposure to asbestos
B   May develop 40 years after exposure to asbestos
C   Usually metastasizes to regional lymph nodes
D   Should be treated by surgical resection
E   Responds to radiotherapy

18. Iron deficiency
A   May occur on a daily iron intake of 1 mg
B   Causes a hypochromic microcytic anaemia
C   Is associated with a low transferrin
D   Is commoner following partial gastrectomy
E   Occurs in thalassaemia

19. Basal cell carcinoma
A   Is the commonest form of skin cancer
B   Usually occurs on the trunk
C   Commonly metastasizes to regional lymph nodes
D   Responds to radiotherapy
E   May be distinguished from squamous cell carcinoma
    by its rapid growth

20. **Legionnaire's disease**
    A   Is a bacterial infection
    B   Is usually diagnosed by isolation of the organism from blood cultures
    C   May cause gastrointestinal symptoms
    D   Is associated with neutropenia
    E   Usually responds to treatment with penicillin

21. **Myaesthenia gravis**
    A   Is an autoimmune disorder
    B   Commonly presents with ophthalmoplegia
    C   Is associated with thymoma
    D   May respond to thymectomy
    E   Responds to oral anticholinesterases

22. **Vasopressin**
    A   Is a polypeptide
    B   Is synthesized in the posterior pituitary
    C   Is released in response to a fall in plasma osmolality
    D   Promotes renal tubular reabsorption of water
    E   Causes smooth muscle relaxation

23. **Patients with scleroderma**
    A   Are usually female
    B   May develop dysphagia
    C   May develop cardiomyopathy
    D   Often suffer from Raynaud's phenomenon
    E   Usually have an underlying malignancy

24. **Uric acid stones**
    A Are the commonest form of renal calculi
    B Are radio-opaque
    C Form more readily in acid urine
    D May dissolve following treatment with sulphin-pyrazone
    E Rarely occur in the absence of clinical gout

25. **In amoebic liver abscess**
    A The right lobe of the liver is most commonly affected
    B Jaundice is a common presenting feature
    C Amoebic cysts may be identified in aspirated pus
    D The chest X-ray is often abnormal
    E Cardiac tamponade is a recognized complication

26. **Villous adenoma**
    A Is the commonest form of colo-rectal polyp
    B Usually occurs in the right side of the colon
    C Often presents with hyponatraemia
    D Rarely becomes malignant
    E Can usually be managed conservatively

27. **BCG vaccine**
    A Is a live vaccine
    B Elicits a cell mediated (type IV) hypersensitivity reaction
    C Should be given by i.m. injection
    D Produces a local skin reaction within 24 hours
    E Should be given to immunosuppressed patients who have no previous history of tuberculosis

28. **The following are characteristic features of polycy-thaemia rubra vera**
    A Leucocytosis
    B Thrombocytosis
    C Decreased blood viscosity
    D Vascular thrombosis
    E Splenomegaly

29. **Parkinson's disease may respond to treatment with**
    A L-dopa
    B Anticholinergic drugs
    C Bromocriptine
    D Reserpine
    E Chlorpromazine

30. **In Takayasu's arteritis (pulseless disease)**
    A Young women are most commonly affected
    B Small and medium sized arteries are usually involved
    C Hypertension is a recognized finding
    D The ESR is usually raised
    E Return of arterial pulses may follow corticosteroid therapy

31. **The following drugs may cause gynaecomastia**
    A Spironolactone
    B Digoxin
    C Levo dopa
    D α methyl dopa
    E Metoclopramide

32. **Homocystinuria**
    A Is inherited as an autosomal recessive
    B Is associated with an increased tendency to thrombosis
    C Is associated with dislocation of the lens of the eye
    D May respond to treatment with pyridoxine
    E Is associated with short stature

33. **The following findings are important in establishing the absence of brainstem function**
    A Fixed dilated pupils
    B Presence of doll's eye movements
    C Absence of cough reflex
    D Absence of spontaneous respiration
    E Iso-electric EEG

34. **Folic acid deficiency**
    A Is common in vegetarians
    B Causes a macrocytic anaemia
    C Occurs in association with terminal ileitis
    D May be caused by phenytoin
    E May occur in haemolytic anaemias

35. **Carbon monoxide**
    A Is the commonest form of self poisoning in the UK
    B Has an affinity for haemoglobin ten times that of oxygen
    C Is an irritant gas
    D Causes cyanosis
    E May cause cerebral infarction

36. **Benign intracranial hypertension**
   A   Is usually associated with dilatation of the ventricles
   B   Rarely causes papilloedema
   C   May cause diplopia
   D   May result in permanent visual loss
   E   May respond to steroids

37. **The following are characteristic of familial vitamin D resistant rickets**
   A   Autosomal recessive inheritance
   B   Low serum phosphate
   C   Low serum calcium
   D   Low levels of vitamin D
   E   Good response to oral 1,25 dihydroxyvitamin D

38. **Giant cell arteritis**
   A   Often presents before the age of 60
   B   Is often associated with a normal ESR
   C   May cause blindness
   D   Usually responds rapidly to steroid therapy
   E   Always requires lifelong treatment

39. **Plasma urea**
   A   Is a more sensitive index of renal function than creatinine
   B   Falls following corticosteroid therapy
   C   Rises following gastrointestinal haemorrhage
   D   Is often low in liver failure
   E   Rises following surgery

40. **In von Willebrand's disease**
   A   Both sexes are equally affected
   B   The partial thromboplastin time is prolonged due to reduced factor VIII clotting activity
   C   Plasma levels of factor VIII-related antigen are increased
   D   Platelet numbers are reduced
   E   The bleeding time is prolonged

41. **The phrenic nerve**
   A   Arises from the 2nd, 3rd and 4th cervical nerves
   B   Carries both afferent and efferent fibres
   C   Is the only motor nerve supply to the diaphragm
   D   Passes behind the root of the lung
   E   Carries sensory fibres from the pericardium

42. **In Q fever endocarditis**
   A   The causative organism is a virus
   B   Blood cultures are sterile
   C   There may be a history of contact with farm animals
   D   Penicillin is the treatment of choice
   E   Treatment should be continued for 6 weeks

43. **In peroneal muscular atrophy**
   A   Inheritance may be X-linked
   B   A predominantly proximal myopathy occurs
   C   There may be a peripheral sensory neuropathy
   D   Wasting of respiratory muscles may occur
   E   Life expectancy is reduced

44. **Eosinophilia may be found in the peripheral blood in**
   A Asthma
   B Polyarteritis nodosa
   C Sarcoid
   D Hodgkin's disease
   E Pulmonary aspergillosis

45. **The following are features of pseudohypoparathyroidism**
   A Hypocalcaemia
   B Raised plasma parathyroid hormone levels
   C Increased urinary cyclic AMP excretion in response
      to i.v. parathyroid hormone
   D Short stature
   E Mental retardation

46. **The following may predispose to the development of
   hepatocellular carcinoma**
   A Hepatitis B virus infection
   B Hepatitis A virus infection
   C Oral contraceptive pill
   D Aflatoxin
   E Haemochromatosis

47. **In hydralazine-induced SLE**
   A Fast acetylators are more likely to be affected
   B Renal involvement is common
   C Resolution rarely occurs on withdrawal of the drug
   D The ANF is usually positive
   E Anti-DNA antibodies are usually present

48. In motor neuron disease
A Men are more commonly affected
B Bulbar palsy may occur
C Sensory signs are usually present
D Muscle weakness and fasciculation occur
E Only lower motor neuron lesions occur

49. Thyroid enlargement may be caused by
A Iodides
B Aspirin
C Phenylbutazone
D Carbimazole
E Para-amino salicylic acid

50. Chondrocalcinosis (pseudogout)
A Is associated with diabetes mellitus
B Is associated with haemochromatosis
C May mimic septic arthritis
D Is associated with radiological calcification within the joint space
E Is associated with the presence of positively bi-refringent crystals in joint effusions

51. The following are characteristic features of retro-peritoneal fibrosis
A Hydronephrosis
B A history of prolonged methysergide ingestion can be obtained in the majority of cases
C Ankle oedema due to vena caval obstruction
D Lateral displacement of the ureters on i.v. pyelography
E Difficulty in performing retrograde pyelography due to obstruction of the passage of ureteric catheters

52. **Cholestatic jaundice of pregnancy**
   A Usually occurs in the first trimester
   B Is rarely associated with pruritus
   C Usually resolves after parturition
   D Rarely recurs in subsequent pregnancies
   E May recur in predisposed women who are given the oral contraceptive pill

53. **Cholecystokinin**
   A Is secreted by the exocrine pancreas
   B Secretion is increased following a protein meal
   C Increases secretion of pancreatic enzymes
   D Causes contraction of the gallbladder
   E Is secreted in excess in coeliac disease

54. **In a coal worker with pneumoconiosis**
   A The chest X-ray may be normal
   B Pulmonary function tests may be normal
   C Massive fibrosis may progress after exposure to coal dust has ceased
   D There may be entitlement to a disability benefit
   E The risk of developing bronchial carcinoma is increased

55. **In glucose-6-phosphate dehydrogenase deficiency**
   A Caucasians are most commonly affected
   B Both sexes are equally affected
   C Red cells may contain Heinz bodies
   D Haemolysis may be precipitated by primaquine
   E Haemolysis may be precipitated by pneumonia

56. Discoid lupus erythematosus
A Is commoner in women
B Is aggravated by sunlight
C Commonly affects the limbs
D May cause alopecia
E Is associated with high titres of anti-DNA antibody

57. Atrial myxoma
A Is the commonest primary intracardiac tumour
B Usually occurs in the right atrium
C May metastasize to regional lymph nodes
D Is associated with clubbing
E May cause sudden death

58. *Clostridium tetanus*
A Produces an exotoxin
B Is a Gram-negative bacillus
C Causes painless muscle spasms
D May cause respiratory muscle paralysis
E Should be treated with tetanus toxoid

59. Patients with Sjögren's syndrome may suffer from
A Corneal ulceration
B Dysphagia
C Recurrent chest infections
D Dyspareunia
E Rheumatoid arthritis

60. Cholesterol gallstones
A Are the commonest form of gallstone
B Are usually radio-opaque
C Are associated with haemolytic anaemia
D Are commoner in women
E May predispose to carcinoma of the gallbladder

ANSWERS

1. DE

In meningococcal meningitis *Neisseria meningitidis* can usually be identified as Gram-negative intracellular diplococci in the CSF and can usually be cultured from blood. The CSF sugar is usually low or absent. Complications may develop rapidly and i.v. penicillin should be started immediately. Prophylactic treatment, usually in the form of rifampicin should be given to close household contacts.

2. BDE

Aldosterone is secreted by the zona glomerulosa of the adrenal cortex and causes renal tubular sodium absorption and potassium loss. Its secretion is controlled by the renin–angiotensin system. Spironolactone competitively inhibits the action of aldosterone on renal tubules.

3. ADE

In phenylketonuria an absence of phenylalanine hydroxylase leads to a reduced conversion of phenylalanine to tyrosine. Detection is by assaying phenylalanine on a heel prick serum. Treatment is with a phenylalanine-free diet and tyrosine supplementation may be required. There is dispute concerning how long the diet should be adhered to, but it is generally accepted that pregnant mothers should return to their diet during pregnancy.

4. A D E

Hyaline casts are composed of Tamm Horsfall protein (uromucoid) which is excreted by normal tubular cells. Cellular casts result from adherence of either red cells (implying glomerular bleeding) or white cells (implying tubular inflammation) to the surface of hyaline casts. Epithelial cells may be found in normal urine due to contamination by cells from the vulva or prepuce. Normal urine contains up to 200 mg protein per day.

5. A D

Gilbert's disease is a familial condition in which there is impaired conjugation of bilirubin and hence acholuria. Bilirubin is raised and is increased by fasting but other liver function tests are normal.

6. A B

In Crohn's disease inflammation tends to be transmural with the mucosa being relatively well preserved. Characteristic granulomata may be found. In ulcerative colitis inflammation is largely mucosal, with depletion of goblet cells and formation of crypt abscesses being characteristic features.

7. B D E

Oat cell carcinoma accounts for about 30% of bronchial carcinoma, the commonest form being squamous cell. Both of these are much commoner in smokers. The tumour is fast growing and has often metastasized at the time of presentation. Ectopic production of ADH and ACTH are common.

8. ACE

Although extensive bone involvement due to malignant plasma cell proliferation is common in myeloma, bone lesions are usually entirely destructive with no demonstrable osteoclastic activity. This is thought to account for the normal alkaline phosphatase. Plasma cells normally constitute 5–10% of the bone marrow population.

9. AD

Ostium secundum atrial septal defects account for 70% of atrial septal defects and rarely cause symptoms before middle age when heart failure may be precipitated by the development of atrial fibrillation. Delayed closure of the pulmonary valve (due to volume overload of the right ventricle) results in wide fixed splitting of the second heart sound. There is usually evidence of partial right bundle branch block, right ventricular hypertrophy and right axis deviation on ECG. Endocarditis due to infection of an ostium secundum defect is very uncommon.

10. ABE

Following subarachnoid haemorrhage, a marked catecholamine release commonly causes glycosuria and ECG changes. Rebleeding is not unusual up to 6 weeks after which the incidence declines. Analgesics which may cause sedation or excessive pupillary changes should be avoided if possible. Xanthochromia is caused by blood pigments released from lysed red cells and may be absent in the early stages.

11. ABCE

Rheumatoid factor is a circulating IgM with activity against the patient's own IgG. Its ability to agglutinate sheep red cells forms the basis of the sheep cell agglutination test (SCAT). It is found in 70–80% of patients with rheumatoid arthritis, 40% with SLE and less frequently in other conditions. High titres correlate with a worse prognosis and a high incidence of systemic complications.

116

12. ACE

Karyotyping in the testicular feminization syndrome reveals an XY sex chromosome complement but the tissues are resistant to the action of androgens. External appearances, including those of the genitalia, are female although pubic and axillary hair is scanty or absent. The gonads are testes which are often intra-abdominal and susceptible to malignant change.

13. ACE

Glucagon is a polypeptide which is secreted by α cells of the Islets of Langerhan. Secretion is increased during fasting and hypoglycaemia. It antagonizes the effects of insulin, increasing blood glucose by stimulating gluconeogenesis and glycogenolysis.

14. ABCDE

Although hypernephroma classically presents with haematuria, loin pain and an abdominal mass, a number of presentations are recognized. Anaemia may result from haematuria and polycythaemia from increased erythropoietin production. Hypercalcaemia may result from parathyroid hormone production by the tumour, and liver function tests may be abnormal in the absence of hepatic metastases through an unknown mechanism. Secondary amyloid may occur and regress following removal of the tumour.

15. AD

Limb girdle muscular dystrophy usually presents between 20 to 40 years progressing to cause severe disability and often death by the age of 50. The cranial muscles are usually spared.

16. B

Parietal cells are located in the body of the stomach and produce intrinsic factor and acid. Acid production is stimulated by gastrin which is secreted by antral G cells and leads to conversion of pepsinogens, secreted by chief cells, to pepsins. In pernicious anaemia parietal cell atrophy results in achlorhydria and malabsorption of vitamin B_{12} due to the absence of intrinsic factor.

17. B

Mesothelioma usually develops in people who are occupationally exposed to asbestos although exposure may be trivial and usually preceeds tumour development by 20 to 40 years. Metastases are rare but surgical resection is usually precluded by chest wall and mediastinal invasion and radiotherapy and chemotherapy are of no proven benefit.

18. ABD

The normal dietary intake of iron is 15–20 mg, approximately 10% of which is absorbed. Acid improves absorption and hence requirements may increase following partial gastrectomy. Transferrin and total iron binding capacity are raised in iron deficiency. Although thalassaemia causes a mircocytic anaemia the serum iron is raised.

19. AD

Basal cell carcinoma accounts for about 70% of cases of skin cancer, usually occurring on the face and developing as an ulcerating nodule which is locally invasive but virtually never metastasizes. Its relatively slow growth helps to distinguish it from squamous cell carcinoma. Local excision or radiotherapy are both effective treatments and usually result in complete cure.

118

20. A C
Legionnaire's disease is caused by a Gram-negative rod (*Legionella pneumophilia*) which is difficult to culture. The diagnosis is usually made by detecting a rising antibody titre. Gastrointestinal and neurological symptoms are common and the white cell count is usually raised with a neutrophilia. Erythromycin, together with rifampicin in severe cases, is the treatment of choice.

21. A B C D E
In myaesthenia gravis, antibodies to acetylcholine receptors in the post-synaptic membrane have been found. Ptosis or diplopia are the usual presenting features and remission may be induced by thymectomy even in the absence of thymoma.

22. A D
Vasopressin is a cyclic octapeptide which is synthesized in the hypothalamic nuclei and passes along the neurohypophyseal tract to the posterior pituitary from which it is released. It promotes renal tubular reabsorption of water and is released in response to a rise in plasma osmolality. If given in pharmacological doses it stimulates smooth muscle contraction but this effect is probably not important physiologically.

23. A B C D
Scleroderma is characterized by widespread and diffuse fibrosis affecting the skin, gastrointestinal tract, heart, skeletal and smooth muscle. Initial swelling of the collagen fibres is followed by fibrosis. Raynaud's phenomenon occurs in over 75% of cases. An association with underlying malignancy is not recognized.

24. C
Radiolucent uric acid stones account for 5–10% of renal calculi. They may occur in the absence of gout, hyperuricaemia or hyperuricosuria (which may be induced by uricosuric drugs such as sulphinpyrazone). The excretion of a persistently acid urine which diminishes uric acid solubility is important.

25. ADE
Amoebic liver abscess usually occurs posteriorly in the right lobe. Jaundice is uncommon. The chest X-ray may reveal an elevated hemidiaphragm, linear atelectasis or shadowing at the right base or an empyema or lung abscess due to rupture into the pleural cavity or lung. Tamponade may result from rupture into the pericardium. Motile amoebae, but not cysts, may be identified in aspirated pus.

26. None
The commonest colo-rectal polyp is a tubular adenoma. Villous adenoma occurs almost exclusively in the rectum and lower sigmoid colon and often presents with hypokalaemia due to potassium losses in mucus and fluid secretions. It has a high malignant potential and surgical resection is always required.

27. AB
Bacille–Calmette–Guerin is a live attenuated strain of tuberculosis and should not be given if immunity is impaired. It is given by intradermal injection and provides a classical example of a cell-mediated hypersensitivity reaction, producing a local skin reaction within 3 to 4 weeks.

28. ABDE

Erythrocytosis in polycythaemia is usually accompanied by an increase in granulocyte and platelet production. Blood viscosity is increased and together with the thrombocytosis predisposes to vascular thromboses. Myeloid metaplasia may occur in the liver and spleen resulting in hepatosplenomegaly. Progression to myelofibrosis is not uncommon.

29. ABC

Treatment of Parkinson's disease is aimed at restoring the balance between the cholinergic and dopaminergic systems in the basal ganglia, the latter being deficient. Bromocriptine is a dopamine agonist but reserpine depletes dopamine stores and chlorpromazine antagonizes dopamine receptors.

30. ACDE

Takayasu's arteritis usually affects the aortic arch and thoracic aorta together with the proximal segments of the large branches. Hypertension may result from renal artery involvement. The ESR is usually raised and systemic symptoms may be present. Corticosteroids are usually effective in management and may result in return of arterial pulses.

31. ABDE

Drugs which act as dopamine antagonists (such as α methyl dopa and metoclopramide) may cause gynaecomastia by increasing prolactin levels. Digoxin binds to oestrogen receptors and has an oestrogenic effect and spironolactone has anti-androgenic properties.

32. ABCD
In homocystinuria, an absence of the enzyme cystathionine synthase, for which pyridoxine is a cofactor, leads to a reduced conversion of homocystine to cytathionine. Homocystine accumulates in plasma and urine. Many of the clinical manifestations are related to abnormal connective tissue. They include ectopia lentis, lax ligaments, osteoporosis, lengthened extremities and mental retardation. Death from thrombosis is not uncommon.

33. ACD
To establish the absence of brainstem function, all brainstem reflexes should be proved to be absent. These include the lack of pupillary and corneal reflexes, absence of eye movements either in response to movements of the head (doll's eye movements) or in response to injection of cold water into the ear (caloric responses), and the absence of laryngeal reflexes and spontaneous respiration. The EEG is less helpful in assessing brainstem function and iso-electric EEG's have been recorded in patients who have subsequently recovered.

34. BDE
Folic acid is found in green vegetables and liver. It is absorbed in the proximal third of the small intestine. Phenytoin interferes with folic acid absorption and metabolism. Requirements are increased by increased red cell formation in haemolytic anaemias.

35. E
The incidence of carbon monoxide poisoning in the UK has fallen dramatically since the advent of 'natural gas'. It has an affinity for haemoglobin 200 times that of oxygen and forms carboxyhaemoglobin which is pink. Carbon monoxide itself is non-irritant but it may be inhaled with fumes that are. Symptoms result from anoxia, and cerebral infarction may occur, particularly in watershed areas.

36. CDE

In benign intracranial hypertension, the CSF pressure is raised in the absence of a space-occupying lesion. The ventricles are usually normal or even reduced in size. Papilloedema and 6th nerve palsies occur. The condition may respond to steroids but in cases with severe papilloedema, surgical decompression of the optic nerve may be required to prevent permanent visual loss.

37. B

Familial vitamin D resistant rickets (familial hypophosphataemic rickets) is a sex-linked dominant disorder. A defect in cellular transport is thought to cause a renal tubular phosphate leak and impaired phosphate absorption. Serum calcium and vitamin D levels are normal and response to oral vitamin D is poor.

38. CD

Giant cell arteritis (originally described as temporal or cranial arteritis) is rare before the age of 60. Inflammation occurs in large and small arteries often with the presence of giant cells. Blindness due to central retinal artery occlusion is common and sudden unilateral blindness in an elderly patient should always raise the possibility of this condition. The ESR is very rarely normal and the response to steroids is usually immediate and dramatic. The disease often burns itself out in 1–2 years when treatment can be gradually withdrawn.

39. CDE

Creatinine is produced at a roughly constant rate, proportional to skeletal muscle mass. In contrast the production rate of urea is much more variable, increasing with increased cellular catabolism (as in infection, trauma or steroid therapy) or following a protein load (either dietary or following gastrointestinal haemorrhage). It may be low in liver failure due to reduced production.

40. ABE

Von Willebrand's disease is an autosomal dominant condition in which there is both factor VIII deficiency and defective platelet function. Factor VIII consists of several components. A low molecular weight portion, factor VIII C, provides the coagulant activity and is deficient in both haemophilia and von Willebrand's disease. A high molecular weight portion, factor VIII-related antigen has no clotting activity but may be recognized immunologically. It is reduced in von Willebrand's disease but normal in haemophilia. Platelet numbers are normal but platelet aggregation is reduced leading to a prolonged bleeding time.

41. BCE

The phrenic nerve arises from 3rd, 4th and 5th cervical nerves. It provides the sole motor supply to the diaphragm. In the thorax it passes in front of the root of the lung, running alongside the pericardium which it supplies. It also carries sensory fibres from the mediastinal pleura, and the pleura and peritoneum covering the diaphragm.

42. BC

Q fever is caused by the rickettsia *Coxiella burneti* which is endemic in cattle and sheep throughout the world. It usually presents as an acute illness with fevers, severe malaise and cough but may cause a chronic endocarditis. The diagnosis is confirmed by a rising antibody titre. Tetracycline is the treatment of choice although the response even to long-term treatment is variable and valve replacement is often required.

124

43. AC
Although peroneal muscular atrophy usually has a dominant inheritance, recessive and X-linked transmission have been described. Degeneration of anterior horn cells, dorsal columns and peripheral nerves results in atrophy of the distal lower limb muscles and, in some cases, a sensory neuropathy. The disorder runs a very slow course and may arrest spontaneously. Wasting is always confined to the limbs and life expectancy is normal.

44. ABDE
Eosinophilia is characteristic of allergic conditions, including asthma and drug reactions, and parasitic infestations. In addition it may indicate a variety of underlying disorders including carcinoma or lymphoma (particularly Hodgkin's disease) and polyarteritis nodosa.

45. ABDE
Pseudohypoparathyroidism is an inherited disorder in which renal and bone receptors fail to respond to parathyroid hormone. Plasma parathyroid hormone levels are raised and urinary cyclic AMP levels fail to rise in response to exogenous parathyroid hormone. In addition to the usual features of hypoparathyroidism, patients often have short stature, shortening of the 4th metacarpal, obesity and mental retardation.

46. ACDE
Although hepatocellular carcinoma is uncommon in Europe, the incidence is much higher in Africa and S.E. Asia. Several possible aetiological factors have been implicated including hepatitis B virus infection and aflatoxin, a toxin derived from the mould *Aspergillus flavus* which may contaminate food. Hepatocellular carcinoma develops in up to 30% of patients with haemochromatosis and rare cases may follow prolonged use of oral contraceptives.

47. D
The development of hydralazine-induced SLE is dose related. Hydralazine is metabolized by acetylation in the liver and the syndrome is therefore more likely to develop in slow acetylators. Renal and CNS involvement are rare. Resolution usually occurs on withdrawal of the drug although this may take months or years. The ANF is invariably positive but DNA antibodies are usually absent.

48. ABD
In motor neuron disease upper and lower motor neuron lesions occur due to degeneration of anterior horn cells, brain-stem nuclei or corticospinal tracts. Men are affected twice as often as women. Sensory loss 'never' occurs.

49. ACDE
Carbimazole, and to a lesser extent phenylbutazone and para-amino salicylates, interfere with production of thyroid hormone resulting in increased secretion of TSH which may cause thyroid enlargement. Iodine itself in excess also interferes with the production and release of thyroid hormone.

50. ABCDE
Chondrocalcinosis, due to calcium pyrophosphate deposition within joints, is associated with diabetes, haemochromatosis and hyperparathyroidism. It may cause an acute arthritis, resembling a septic arthritis, but the diagnosis may be confirmed by finding radiological calcification of the joint capsule and cartilage and positively birefringent crystals of calcium pyrophosphate in the joint effusion.

51. AC

In retroperitoneal fibrosis the ureters become embedded in dense fibrous tissue resulting in ureteric obstruction and hydronephrosis. The vena cava may also be involved. The aetiology is unknown in over 50% of cases but retroperitoneal malignancy, particularly lymphoma, and prolonged methysergide therapy may be implicated in the remainder. Characteristic radiological findings are medial displacement of the ureters and ease of passage of ureteric catheters despite functional obstruction.

52. CE

Benign intrahepatic cholestasis may occur in some women during pregnancy, usually in the third trimester. Pruritus is usually the presenting feature and may be severe. The cholestasis characteristically resolves rapidly following parturition but commonly recurs in subsequent pregnancies or in predisposed women who are given oral contraceptive steroids.

53. BCD

Cholecystokinin is produced in the small intestine in response to the presence of fat or amino acids. Production may therefore be reduced if the small intestinal mucosa is abnormal. It stimulates pancreatic secretion and gallbladder contraction.

54. BCD

Coal worker's pneumoconiosis is diagnosed radiologically and classified according to the size of pulmonary nodules. In massive fibrosis lesions larger than 1 cm diameter are present and progression occurs even after exposure to coal dust has ceased. Pulmonary function tests may be normal in simple pneumoconiosis but become abnormal as massive fibrosis develops. Disability benefits may be awarded to sufferers by the Pneumoconiosis Board of the Department of Health. There is no evidence that pneumoconiosis predisposes to the development of bronchial carcinoma.

55. CDE
Glucose-6-phosphate dehydrogenase deficiency is an incompletely dominant sex-linked disorder which is common in Africa, the Mediterranean and Middle and Far East. Haemolysis may be induced by oxidant drugs (such as primaquine) or acute infections. One factor implicated in the development of haemolysis is the increased tendency of haemoglobin to be oxidized to methaemoglobin, being further precipitated as Heinz bodies.

56. ABD
Discoid lupus erythematosus most commonly affects the face and scalp. The well defined, erythematous, scaling lesions are exacerbated by sunlight and cause scarring which results in irreversible alopecia on affected areas of scalp. Unlike systemic lupus erythematosus, lesions are confined to the skin and although ANF may be present the anti-DNA antibody titre is usually low.

57. ADE
Atrial myxoma accounts for about 50% of primary intracardiac tumours (all of which are rare) usually occurring on the left. It is benign but may present with constitutional effects such as fever, weight loss, anaemia, clubbing and raised ESR. Left atrial myxoma may prolapse into and obstruct the mitral valve and may embolize into the systemic circulation.

58. AD
Clostridium tetanus is a Gram-positive spore-forming bacillus. It produces an exotoxin which is toxic to the CNS causing painful muscle spasms and paralysis which often involve respiratory muscles. Tetanus toxoid is used to prevent tetanus but not in acute attacks which should be treated with tetanus immunoglobulin to neutralize the toxin, surgical debridement of an infected wound and penicillin to eradicate existing infection.

59. A B C D E
Sjögren's syndrome consists of keratoconjunctivitis sicca (dry eyes leading in some cases to corneal ulceration) and xerostomia (dry mouth), usually with a connective tissue disorder (most commonly rheumatoid arthritis). Secretions from lachrymal and salivary glands are reduced and other epithelial surfaces such as the trachea and bronchi, oesophagus and vagina may be affected.

60. A D E
Cholesterol gallstones are the commonest form of gallstones and are commoner in women. They do not usually contain calcium and are thus radio-lucent. In chronic haemolysis, increased bilirubin production may lead to the development of pigment rather than cholesterol gallstones. Carcinoma of the gallbladder is a rare complication of gallstones.